EARLY DETECTION

Kirsten E. Gardner

EARLY
DETECTION

WOMEN,

CANCER, &

AWARENESS

CAMPAIGNS

IN THE

TWENTIETH-

CENTURY

UNITED

STATES

The University of
North Carolina Press
CHAPEL HILL

Designed by Heidi Perov
Set in Cycles

Manufactured in the United States of America

This volume was published with the generous
assistance of the Greensboro Women's Fund of the
University of North Carolina Press. Founding Contributors:
Linda Arnold Carlisle, Sally Schindel Cone, Anne Faircloth,
Bonnie McElveen Hunter, Linda Bullard Jennings, Janice J.
Kerley (in honor of Margaret Supplee Smith), Nancy Rouzer
May, and Betty Hughes Nichols.

The paper in this book meets the guidelines for permanence
and durability of the Committee on Production Guidelines
for Book Longevity of the Council on Library Resources.

Library of Congress Cataloging-in-Publication Data
Gardner, Kirsten E. (Kirsten Elizabeth)
    Early detection : women, cancer, and awareness campaigns
in the twentieth-century United States / Kirsten E. Gardner.
        p. cm.
Includes bibliographical references and index.
    ISBN-13: 978-0-8078-3014-7 (cloth: alk. paper)
    ISBN-10: 0-8078-3014-3 (cloth: alk. paper)
    ISBN 13: 978-0-8078-5682-6 (pbk.: alk. paper)
    ISBN 10: 0-8078-5682-7 (pbk.: alk. paper)
    1. Cancer in women—Social aspects—History—20th
century. 2. Cancer in women—Political aspects—
History—20th century. I. Title.
    RC281.W65G37   2006
    362.196'9940082—dc22   2005035577

cloth   10 09 08 07 06   5 4 3 2 1
paper   10 09 08 07 06   5 4 3 2 1

Dedicated in memory of my mother,
Christine Eisenhardt Gardner, 1946–1996

Contents

Figures and Illustrations

Acknowledgments

This book started as a dissertation at the University of Cincinnati, where I was fortunate to work with outstanding faculty in history and women's studies. My mentor, Joanne Meyerowitz, patiently awaited drafts of my chapters and readily offered insight, advice, and guidance. She is an inspirational scholar, and I thank her for her wisdom and friendship. Roger Daniels worked with me on this project for many years, sending advice from around the globe while on various sabbaticals. He continues to encourage and critique. I appreciate time spent with him, which is always a learning experience. Barbara Ramusack served on my dissertation committee, encouraging me throughout the process. As I pursued this topic, I learned immeasurably from historians of medicine. In particular, Barron Lerner served as an outside reader on my dissertation committee and has consistently impressed me with his generosity, kind spirit, collaborative impulse, and keen intellect.

At the University of Cincinnati the Taft Fellowship, University Graduate Scholarship, and History Department Travel Funds provided important financial support for this project. I also participated in the Future Faculty Seminar at the University of Cincinnati under the guidance of Howard Jackson, and his energy and devotion to teaching better prepared me for life at the University of Texas at San Antonio.

Archivists and librarians have helped me throughout this project. In particular, I am grateful for their assistance at the Library of Congress Manuscript Division, the American Association of University Women Archives, the General Federation of Women's Clubs Archives, the National Archives and Records Administration, and the Grand Lodge of Cedar Rapids, Iowa.

Over the years I have been surrounded by wonderful and encouraging friends, colleagues, and family. Thank you to each and every one of you. In particular, thanks to my father, sisters, and brothers. I lived with my family during the initial years of this project, and in addition to meals, housing, and continual sounds of laughter, they provided an environment conducive to my work and studies. I could not have completed this without the support of my father, Neal Gardner, Brother Neal's encouragement, Bridget's public health expertise, long walks with Megan, Tobin's musical distractions, and hours with Caitlin sitting patiently by my side, helping with notes and citations, and always confident that this book would reach completion. My mother, Christine, died from breast cancer as this project was forming in my mind. Although she is not here physically, her spirit and memory offer a constant source of inspiration.

Friends and colleagues have read various chapters of this work, graciously sharing their time and insight. In particular, thank you to Susan Freeman, Shelley McKellar, Emilie Johnson, Gregg Michel, Gaye Theresa Johnson, Rhonda Gonzales, Patrick Kelly, Kolleen Guy, and Anne Hardgrove. Additionally, scholars working on cancer, including David Cantor, Barron Lerner, Leslie Reagan, and participants of the Annecy Cancer Program, have shared ideas, useful suggestions, and advice at critical moments in this project. Several graduate students assisted with research. Special thanks to Patrick Murphy and Andria Crossen.

The University of Texas at San Antonio has also supported this work with the COLFA summer research fund and the University Faculty Research Award. It has been a pleasure to work with my editor, Sian Hunter, throughout this publishing process. Several readers offered valuable suggestions for this manuscript. I particularly thank Susan L. Smith and Emily Abel. Thanks also to the University of North Carolina Press staff and anonymous readers.

Finally, Buddy Baron has spent more time by my side than I deserve throughout these past several years. His companionship is treasured daily.

EARLY DETECTION

Introduction

I started my research on breast cancer in the early 1990s. Then, my research was personal. Doctors had just diagnosed my mother with stage III breast cancer, and I searched for answers to the medical questions that deluge anyone learning of such a diagnosis. The information available to me, my mother, and family members was remarkable. Contemporary magazines featured intelligent articles on breast cancer. Films, radio programs, the Internet, and television shows explained the behavior of the disease and the choices for treatment. My mother was fortunate enough to have access to medical care, and the doctors met with us frequently to discuss the diagnosis, explain test results, and outline treatment options. We analyzed a wealth of information presented by the media, medical community, and cancer activists.

The amount of public attention directed to women and cancer has only increased since then. In the twenty-first century, breast cancer is a public and political issue that is evident throughout American culture. Breast cancer survivors and activists make their personal experiences with the disease public, speaking about their cancer experience at conventions, marches, walks, medical gatherings, and community meetings. Likewise, publications about women and cancer have multiplied in recent years, and the content of publications ranges from intimate reflections on illness to medical definitions and theories.[1] Since 1991, the breast cancer survivors and activists who formed the National Breast Cancer Coalition (NBCC), one of the most powerful lobbying groups for women's health in the country, have directed increased political attention to women and cancer.[2] While scientists and activists argue about the rate of breast cancer incidence, note the lack of public funds earmarked for female diseases, and compare the consequences of different detection and treatment options, the media tries to convey this information to a lay audience. Politicians also engage in the debate, and by the 1990s political analysts recognized support for breast cancer research as an emerging issue in voting behavior. As journalist Gina Kolata wrote, "Forget the deficit. Forget taxes. Forget Medicare. Politicians, hoping to appeal to women, are now engaged in the battle of the breast."[3]

As part of this contemporary public discourse, breast cancer activists, government officials, and media reporters have often alluded to a history of silence, passivity, and neglect that surrounds this disease. Perhaps as a way of emphasizing the importance of an open discussion about women's health and the risk of cancer, spokespersons stress, by way of contrast, the current visibility of breast cancer. As the NBCC explains, the organization "refused to be defeated by the conspiracy of silence and indifference" surrounding breast cancer. In the early 1990s Secretary of Health and Human Services Donna Shalala asserted that the NBCC had "transformed breast cancer from a closely guarded secret—an issue once considered unfit for polite conversation—and brought the issue to the front pages of our newspapers, to the frontsteps of American households, and to the front burner of the national agenda."[4] The press has reinforced this version of history, in which present publicity replaces past silence. Canadian journalist Sharon Batt pointed to "a rapid evolution of women with breast cancer—from passive optimists to impatient activists."[5] In 2002 Natalie Angier wrote, "Not very long ago, the word 'cancer' was a verbal anvil, flattening all nuance, sense and hope. Doctors didn't tell patients; family members didn't tell friends."[6]

As a modern U.S. historian reading these narratives of silence, I became curious about the social and cultural history surrounding women and cancer in America. Familiar with the radical changes ushered in by the feminist health movement, I wondered how women negotiated health decisions prior to the 1970s. Did women know about cancer's biological behavior and the science that explained it? When did they learn about breast self-examinations? Did patients understand the benefits and risks of treatment? Did women with cancer discuss their situation with physicians, family, and friends? I started to research the public discussions of cancer in the early decades of the twentieth century as a way to better understand the complicated reality surrounding women and cancer today.

My research revealed that these frequent references to a "history of silence" obscure a rich history of women's participation in cancer awareness programs since the early 1900s. As historian Barbara Clow has recently argued about the early twentieth century, "Although many people shrank from a frank discussion of the disease as well as knowledge of a devastating diagnosis, their reticence was not absolute, as implied by the term 'silence.' In a variety of ways and for a number of reasons, doctors, sufferers, and the general public were frequently prepared to read, write, and talk about cancer."[7] This book contributes to emerging scholarship that recognizes the legacy of cancer activism, defined as participation in and promotion of cancer awareness programs, in modern history. American women supported cancer educational programs, through both financial contributions and voluntary participation, throughout the twentieth century. Since 1913 and the creation of the American Society for the Control of Cancer (ASCC), women have promoted cancer control by learning about the disease and securing funds for cancer education and research.

Women involved in cancer as a public health project also contributed to broader social trends in the history of medicine. They advanced a professional agenda that placed licensed physicians at the center of cancer treatment and endorsed their medical theories that emphasized the significance of cancer detection. My work traces the twentieth-century history of women's participation in cancer control efforts throughout the United States. I examine the history of the ASCC, public health information on cancer, and popular sources of cancer education, which reveal a history of female involvement and support for cancer awareness. Although much of my focus is on breast and cervical cancer, I examine how women have discussed various cancers specific to their sex, including cancers of the breast, cervix, ovary, and uterus.

When I started this project, I hoped that a historical inquiry would begin to explain why recent literature on breast cancer is so accessible and why publications prior to the 1970s seemed very small in number and narrow in scope. I assumed the dearth of information prior to 1970 reflected the aforementioned history of "silence." I imagined that my work would explore the limited public information about the disease, especially in the pre–World War II era. I thought my sources would recount individual experiences as recorded in diaries and letters. Instead, as I pursued this project, I moved away from individual accounts of cancer and elected to explore mass publications and educational literature produced throughout the twentieth century. Although I found the former insightful and fascinating, I discovered a clearer historical pattern in the printed record that told a rich story of women's contributions to cancer awareness programs in dominant American culture.

My research indicates that the dramatic publicity in recent years stems from a long legacy of women's participation in cancer control. Throughout the twentieth century, hundreds of thousands of women volunteered their time and energy to inform other women about cancer. Private meetings, public viewings of cancer educational films, and informative articles in popular magazines were some of the many ways that women learned about breast and reproductive cancers throughout the twentieth century.

By focusing on the role of women as cancer educators and the impact of women's clubs and voluntary associations in this public health campaign throughout the twentieth century, I argue that contemporary public dialogue about cancer has been informed by a history of women's concerns about breast and reproductive cancer. Many of the twentieth-century cancer education campaigns targeted women, urged women to be vigilant about early detection of cancer, and fostered a sense of optimism about the disease. When *Ladies' Home Journal* asked its readers, "What Can We Do about Cancer?" in 1913, it conveyed details about women and cancer incidence, instruction about detection, and definitions of treatment options and stressed that early detection offered a key for curing cancer. As women learned this information, they often conveyed it to broader female audiences through club meetings, volunteer work, and street booth displays. Early publications issued by the ASCC also taught women about cancer. Printed in several languages, these pamphlets, distributed by female volunteers to diverse immigrant populations throughout the United States, urged women to look for lumps in their breasts and irregular vaginal discharge. As early as the 1920s, women viewed silent educational films with plots that featured women with cancer. A decade later the emerging network of women engaged in cancer awareness programs became more evident as women's clubs throughout the United States, led by the American Association of University Women, organized to educate each other about cancers particular to their sex. One such campaign, organized around a concern for cervical cancer, circulated a manifesto in 1931 entitled *The Protection of Women from Cancer: An Educational Program by Women, for Women, with Women*, reflecting a burgeoning feminist consciousness evident in many of these efforts.[8]

In sum, since the early decades of the twentieth century, women have participated in educational programs that were designed to teach the public about cancer risks, warning signs, and incidence. Throughout much of the twentieth century, they cooperated with medical experts and without question advanced conventional medical opinion about women and cancer treatment. Women's clubs and female associations hosted countless cancer programs, regularly exporting the message of early detection. Indeed, public cancer awareness programs relied on gendered notions of cooperative women who deferred to medical authority. This book examines how, over time, women contributed to popular knowledge about female cancers, often legitimizing medical messages that insisted that early detection worked. Although women's participation in cancer control efforts changed over time, throughout the twentieth century women informed popular notions of cancer. Those involved in cancer awareness encouraged other women to become familiar with their bodies and respond to "cancer warning signs."

In the early twentieth century cancer control was a particular concern for women. First, dominant culture and gendered norms dictated that women should take care of the family and be aware of health dangers.[9] These cultural norms facilitated cancer education programs that targeted women and taught them the seven major warning signs of cancer. Designed by medical professionals, this conventional cancer message urged audiences to react immediately to any warning signs by consulting, and urging family members to consult, medical experts. Moreover, because women's susceptibility to breast and reproductive cancers placed them in a high-risk category, twentieth-century cancer educators emphasized the importance of early detection for women (and this message still resonates today). Urging women to conduct breast self-examinations and have routine vaginal smears (beginning in the 1950s), cancer awareness advocates insisted that if women detected cancer early, then physicians would be able to cure it. Until recent decades, women publicized these conventional medical ideas without challenging them.

By the end of the century, women objected to the insinuations of blame associated with the dominant message of early and self-detection, challenged the orthodoxy of early detection and screening technology, criticized radical treatment, and questioned the absence of female patients' voices in medical doctrine. Moreover, in the twenty-first century, women have radically reframed early education programs to include discussions of treatment alternatives and choices, postsurgical concerns, and issues of sexuality and identity. Contemporary and effective political activism demands greater governmental support for women and cancer.

How did cancer, especially breast cancer, become such a public and political topic? Part of that answer can be found in this history that traces women's contributions to cancer education. Women have promoted early detection, secured funds for cancer control, publicized cancer warning signs, encouraged women to participate in cancer awareness, questioned screening techniques, and most recently challenged conventional treatment norms. This book explores women's participation in cancer control, as educators, organizers, and activists throughout the twentieth century. It reviews the historical emphasis on early detection and the programs that promoted it. Early detection has become pervasive in dominant American culture, advancing a monolithic paradigm for controlling cancer. The message of early detection continues to advance claims that curing cancer is largely dependent on the stage of diagnosis and thereby ignites hope that meticulous screening can ward off a late stage diagnosis. This paradigm influences women's lives in particular. Despite many critical reviews of modern screening technology, most believe that cervical screening and mammography offer women a better means to early detection.[10] This book recalls the legacy of early detection programs as a way to recognize the great strides of this education campaign but also as a way to create space where the merits of early detection rhetoric can be reconsidered in the twenty-first century. As cancer activists have noted, cancer control is about more than early detection. What are the environmental causes of cancer? How should society balance quality of life issues with aggressive cancer cure efforts? How should Americans consider cancers that cannot currently be controlled or cured? How can health efforts include marginalized communities who often lack access to cancer screening technology?

This book contributes to the growing field of scholarship on the history of cancer that examines this dreaded disease within its social and cultural context. Several scholars have already examined the broader history of cancer. Daniel De Moulin's succinct 1983 study, *A Short History of Breast Cancer*, offers a thorough synopsis of the medical history of breast cancer from antiquity to the modern era. *The Dread Disease: Cancer and Modern American Culture* (1987) by James Patterson examines popular understandings of and federal policy regarding cancer within the social and cultural context of twentieth-century U.S. history. More recently, Barron Lerner's *The Breast Cancer*

Wars: Hope, Fear, and the Pursuit of a Cure in Twentieth-Century America (2001) offers insightful analysis of historical trends in the detection, diagnosis, and treatment of breast cancer. He demonstrates how new standards of care gradually evolved in response to patient experiences and demands.

Public health experts, environmentalists, sociologists, and other specialists have also contributed to an emerging field of inquiry about the history of female cancer in modern America. Ellen Leopold's *The Darker Ribbon* (1999) presents a critical review of medical care that tended to objectify female patients. Karen Stabiner's *To Dance with the Devil: The New War on Breast Cancer* (1997) traces the experiences of several patients in the University of California, Los Angeles, comprehensive breast cancer center and its innovative treatment. *Negotiating Disease: Power and Cancer Care, 1900–1950* (2001) by Barbara Clow offers useful and insightful historical analysis on unconventional cancer treatments. Like Clow, I argue that patients learned about cancer through a variety of sources in the twentieth century. In particular, my work examines how American women learned much of their information about cancer from other women. Recent works have made important strides in expanding our knowledge of cancer in the twentieth century, yet we still have much to learn about the role of health intermediaries who parlayed information from professional to lay audiences. In the early twentieth century women began to participate in cancer awareness and served as liaisons between the medical profession and the lay communities it served.[11]

This account contributes to recent scholarship by tracing women's involvement in several activist organizations of the twentieth century. The story is framed by the efforts of the American Society for the Control of Cancer, which evolved into the American Cancer Society (ACS) in 1945. The largest cancer society in the world, it originally envisioned women as the subjects of an educational campaign. Soon after its creation, however, it recruited women to launch cancer awareness programs and to promote early detection. The ASCC originated in New York City as a dream of male medical professionals. The ASCC, and later the ACS, maintained its male leadership, but it quickly welcomed women to the society. Although the ACS stated ambitious goals of educating the entire U.S. population, until recent decades many of its educational efforts targeted an audience that reflected its membership, white citizens with higher education levels, class status, and access to health care. I analyze the ASCC/ACS publications, films, and programs as a way to examine how this organization influenced dominant American culture and its portrayal of cancer. The book traces how female cancer activists both reinforced and challenged this trend over time.

Next, I explore the role of women's clubs as forums for female cancer education, especially places for cancer awareness programs from the 1930s through the 1960s. Lectures, pamphlets, and letters issued and distributed by these clubs emphasized women's need for regular medical exams and urged women to demand routine cancer screenings from their physicians. The women's clubs fostered dialogue about female health concerns and used all-female venues to facilitate open discussions of cancer. A wide range of women's clubs participated in cancer awareness, including organizations of working-class women, women of color, and university women.

I also examine the role of the federal government. Today, the government is the largest contributor to medical research, and contemporary pressure to fund research on women and cancer has manifested in interesting ways, including the distribution of hundreds of millions of dollars for breast cancer research through the Department of Defense.[12] Women have played critical roles in directing more funds to female cancers. Finally, I report and analyze some testimony of women affected by female cancers in this era. I do not attempt to give a representative sample or overview of women's voices but instead use their words to fill certain gaps in the written record and to recognize the personal dimensions of this disease in so many people's lives. Medical records, oral interviews, and autobiographies reflect how women perceived the disease at different historical moments and how their image of breast or reproductive cancer was shaped by the social and cultural context in which they lived.

Texts, visual images, and films produced throughout the twentieth century offer additional information about public awareness of cancer in the early decades of this century. I examined popular magazine articles that the *Readers' Guide to Periodical Literature* indexed under cancer, women's health, breast, uterine, cervical, or ovarian cancer. The public discussion has increased consistently throughout much of the twentieth century. With a few notable exceptions, including the World War II years and the mid-1960s, magazines allotted more space to cancer over time, particularly to cancer and women. I also examined more than twenty educational films about cancer, ranging from ten-minute animated dramas to sixty-minute documentaries. The content of these films varied from technical "how to" advice such as *The Breast Self-Examination* (1949) to dramatic stories of lifesaving decisions such as *Time and Two Women* (1957). The printed material I examined included health pamphlets, educational instructions, posters, and written correspondence.

Finally, certain individuals proved to be movers and shakers in the history of female cancer awareness, continually appearing in a variety of sources and circumstances. These individuals included actuarial expert Frederick Hoffman (1865–1946);[13] doctors Joseph Bloodgood (1867–1935), Arthur Erskine (1885–1952), and George Papanicolaou (1883–1962);[14] activists Florence Becker (1878–1969) and Mary Lasker (1900–1994); and celebrities such as Betty Ford (b. 1918).[15] These individuals get more attention in this study not only because of the important roles they played in educating women about cancer but also because the historical record and archives that hold their private papers provide sources to chronicle their lives and influence on cancer awareness.

In the first half of the twentieth century, women feared breast cancer in the same vein that they feared "generative organ cancers." The popular literature on cancer often failed to specify a certain type of cancer, and when it did, it often referred to "women's cancers" as a subheading that could include both breast and reproductive cancers. Moreover, many women learned about breast and reproductive cancers at the same time, often perceiving "female cancers" as a single category.[16] (Until the introduction of the Pap smear, reproductive cancers had higher mortality figures for women than breast cancer.)[17] When I refer to "female cancers," I am referring to the four major cancers that overwhelmingly occur in females: cancer of the breast, cervix, ovary, and uterus. Although there are hundreds of varieties of cancers, dozens of these cancers primarily affect women, and most of these originate in the breast or reproductive organs.[18]

Chapter 1 introduces the formation of the ASCC and begins to explore women's role as cancer educators in the early decades of the twentieth century. As infectious diseases became less threatening, cancer became a leading cause of death. The ASCC, its physicians, and women volunteers engaged in cancer education that targeted female audiences with hopes that mothers would then convey this information to their families.[19] Since 1987, when James Patterson published his foundational work, *The Dread Disease*, scholars have interrogated the various roles that individuals, institutions, and the government have played in shaping the public perception of cancer. Women played a critical role in creating and promulgating the message of early detection. They fostered a cultural familiarity with cancer among female audiences and urged women to cooperate with medical guidelines for cancer control. The first chapter examines women's willingness to interact with the public, to spread the ASCC's message, and to secure funds that would ensure the organization's survival. Women involved in the ASCC endorsed cancer narratives that stressed early detection; they disseminated medical findings that emphasized the seven warning signs to lay audiences; and they encouraged the government to respond to concerns about cancer.

Chapter 2 is devoted entirely to women's clubs. Female cancer educators correctly imagined that women's clubs, many with membership in the General Federation of Women's Clubs, could act as networks to distribute information on female health issues. They urged women's groups to convey cancer awareness to their large female audiences. Most major women's groups of this era endorsed cancer awareness campaigns, indicating a common concern for cancer among women. My study of women's clubs highlights the importance of dialogue among women in female cancer awareness programs and the role women played as educators in this movement. The activities of the American Association of University Women and the Women's Field Army offer illustrative examples of how noteworthy this movement had become by the late 1930s. Confident that the disease could be controlled more effectively with public education, women, by the hundreds and thousands, advanced an educational campaign that emphasized the importance of early detection and treatment. Women thus contributed to a lasting and perhaps overly optimistic impression that cancer could be controlled with early detection.

The success of early cancer awareness programs cultivated a social sense of concern for women's health, but it also relied on notions of individual responsibility. Women learned to look for cancer symptoms in their own bodies as instructions for self-examination became more clearly defined. Chapter 3 examines the promotion of the breast self-examination, the evolution of the vaginal smear, and the use of films to teach early detection techniques. The emphasis on individual behavior, in an era of postwar hopes and dreams, implied that science offered cancer detection tools that women needed to use effectively. Popular periodicals continued to print articles about cancer, and the content and breadth of the articles were expanded. Autobiographical narratives detailed women's emotional responses to cancer, and the concept of a "cancer survivor" became more common. Often, these personal narratives by women with cancer mirrored the themes of cancer awareness. For instance, many authors recorded stories that highlighted the success of women who detected cancers "early enough" to save their lives. Similarly, cancer education literature, films, and programs underscored success stories by comparing them to alternative versions about women who ignored early symptoms of the disease and ultimately died. Cancer awareness, then, empowered patients with education but also fostered a sense of blaming the victim. To be sure, by the late 1930s the government had become intimately involved in cancer research, as evidenced by the creation of the National Cancer Institute in 1937. World War II created the impetus for further government funding for cancer and much other research related to health, science, and technology. The scientific innovations ushered in by war proved to be a critical turning point in the history of cancer and offered some support to research initiatives that served women.[20]

Chapter 4 explores the expansion and diffusion of information about female cancers at midcentury that often reinforced notions of female domesticity. Although dependent on narrow definitions of womanhood, a formal community of female breast cancer survivors emerged, who consciously recognized shared concerns among women who had been treated for breast cancer. Breast cancer survivor Terese Lasser founded Reach to Recovery in 1954 as a support network for recently diagnosed breast cancer patients. Many of the themes of breast cancer survival reinforced traditional notions of domesticity and stressed the visual importance of the female breast in American culture. I examine the impact of this program and others in the postwar era, which cultivated a consciousness among survivors while also reinforcing conservative gender norms. I also trace the emergence of the breast prosthetic industry, through a brief business history, that demonstrates an economic response to the increasingly self-conscious community of survivors.[21] As recent scholarship demonstrates, the "June Cleaver" image of women in the 1950s is limited and does not reflect a universal experience for women in this era.[22] Cancer educators blurred the boundaries of domesticity, co-opting it for educational purposes, but also subverting it by assuming leadership positions—characteristics that were especially evident among the women's clubs that supported the educational effort and by the activism of women such as Mary Lasker. Chapter 4 also focuses on the transformation of the public discourse on cancer treatment to include more discussion of the pain associated with cancer treatment, the effects of surgery, and the fears of recurrence.

The final chapter recognizes the legacy of women's support for early detection programs. After decades of promulgating the message of early detection, women had ensured that most cancer prevention initiatives would focus on teaching the public about common indications of cancer. Yet, as feminists complained in the late 1960s and 1970s, the medical establishment often treated female patients as passive subjects who should unquestionably comply with the advice of male authorities. Moreover, critics noted, public discussions of cancer erased issues of race and class from the discourse on early detection. Although African American activists had continually worked to promote cancer awareness within the black community, throughout most of the twentieth century, cancer education targeted a white and middle-class audience. To be sure, in the 1930s and 1940s Alice B. Crutcher served as the cancer control chairman of the Federation of Colored Women's Clubs of Kentucky and organized one of the first "Colored Divisions" of the American Cancer Society.[23] By the 1960s the National Council of Negro Women had joined the ACS in its "Conquer Uterine Cancer Now" program. But until recently, most organized cancer awareness programs failed to direct attention to issues of race, class, and ethnicity in a meaningful way.[24]

This final chapter also explores the impact of cancer diagnosis in celebrities. First Lady Betty Ford served as a pioneer in making the personal more political in the crucial decade of the 1970s. Soon after learning that she might have breast cancer, she decided to share her medical diagnosis with the public. A brief survey of the thousands of letters sent to Ford after her diagnosis reveals some of the sentiments that women shared in the early 1970s about breast cancer. As Ford exposed her personal experiences, she lobbied for changes in women's health care and ultimately influenced the public discussions of female cancer and the promotion of mammography.[25] This chapter also examines the implications of female cancer control and the merits of screening technology in an era when feminists politicized the body as a site for empowerment and demanded more accountability from the government and medical profession about women's health issues. The popularity of books that focused on women's health, such as *Our Bodies, Ourselves*, offers one record of the emerging feminist concerns about health.

In recent decades women's historians have explored in great detail the central role that women's clubs, women's networks, and female spaces played in creating more political power for women in the nineteenth and early twentieth centuries and their influence on temperance, woman suffrage, antislavery work, and more.[26] Less attention has been paid to the clubs of the twentieth century and the role that women's clubs played in transforming knowledge about women's health. This book argues that the impact of the feminist health movement can be better appreciated if the participation of women in grassroots educational agendas of earlier decades is recognized. As historians are beginning to note, the "history of silence" is a better indication of the dearth of historical studies about women's participation in cancer campaigns of the early twentieth century than of a lack of women's consciousness in this era.[27] Although cancer activists were not talking about the disease in the early decades of the twentieth century in the ways that patients wanted and needed to talk about it by the century's end, they fostered a discourse about cancer throughout the period.

This book begins to expose the rich legacy of female participation in cancer awareness in modern America. It focuses on women's involvement in grassroots campaigns that were created to educate the public and often emphasized the value of early detection and treatment. It pushes us to consider how notions of progress—the shift from "silence" to publicity—obscure notable historical efforts that urged women to learn more about cancer and its symptoms. *Early Detection* recognizes the important contributions of women invested in cancer control and explores the reasons that the collective memory of these early education programs has been lost.

1

Look Cancer Straight in the Face

PUBLIC DISCUSSIONS OF WOMEN'S CANCERS
IN THE EARLY TWENTIETH CENTURY

In January 1914 dozens of volunteers throughout the northeastern United States distributed a small four-page pamphlet printed by the American Society for the Control of Cancer (ASCC). *Facts about Cancer* may have startled recipients with its frank discussion. The pamphlet immediately stated that sooner or later one in eight women and one in twelve men over the age of thirty-five would succumb to the disease. Moreover, it told readers that cancer did not respect race, religion, or class and it was second only to tuberculosis "as a cause of death and a scourge of the human race." This information likely reinforced dreaded images of cancer. Yet, embedded within this discourse of devastation were messages of hope. The pamphlet insisted that cancer, the common enemy of all persons, could be "EASILY CURED" when recognized and treated in its early stages. Education, it said, could transform the outcome for those cancer victims. By recognizing the illness at its earliest stages and seeking immediate treatment, patients could avoid dying "solely because of ignorance and negligence." By disseminating the pamphlet, these volunteers hoped to decrease cancer mortality.[1]

Americans who resided beyond the northeastern states heard similar messages. Millions of women, to give one example, opened their May 1913 issue of *Ladies' Home Journal* to learn that they could play an important part in controlling cancer.[2] A bold headline proclaimed, "What Can We Do about Cancer?" Taking a cue from the ASCC, author Samuel Hopkins Adams summarized the "best medical advice and opinion on cancer" for female readers: "No cancer is hopeless when discovered early. Most cancer, discovered early, is curable. The only cure is the knife. Medicines are worse than useless. Delay is more than dangerous; it is deadly. The one hope, and a strong one, is prompt and radical operation; a half-operation is worse than none at all."[3] Echoing the sentiments of cancer specialists, Adams stressed the dangers of the disease and the threat of "quacks" who promised to cure it with medicine. As Adams emphasized, early diagnosis offered the only key to the cure.[4]

Throughout the early twentieth century, public health messages such as these provided women and men with information about cancer. The leading medical specialists who created the ASCC in 1913 advocated public education campaigns that taught audiences about the usefulness of cancer detection. They sought ways to ensure that early detection would assume a primary place in twentieth-century efforts to promote health, and they urged the public to cooperate in this professional project. Emerging in the midst of the "new public health" movement, which was informed by Progressive notions that reform organizations could improve society and endorsed by physicians who were interested in medical professionalization, early detection rhetoric suggested that simple behavior modification would contribute to the control of cancer.[5]

This chapter examines the role that women played in the emerging cancer awareness effort. Because cancer educators targeted a female audience, it also analyzes the role of gender in these early twentieth-century education campaigns. Female educators created a common public discourse for cancer, fostered a communal identity among women as an "at-risk" population, introduced terms and ideas that associated notions of hope and optimism with this deadly disease, and raised financial contributions for the society. Hundreds of women participated in this educational agenda at a grassroots level, and in doing so they influenced Americans to fear cancer less and confront it more. Like efforts to end tuberculosis, validate the science of motherhood, and create public knowledge about germ theory, the rise of cancer control reflected changes in medicine whereby medical experts generated knowledge that both shaped and was shaped by women's lives.[6]

The ASCC was committed to educating the public that doctors could treat cancer in its earliest stages. Gaining the support of organized medical groups, including the American Medical Association and the American College of Surgeons, the ASCC created a formal space for those eager to advance cancer control. Despite its overwhelming white, male, and middle- to upper-class leadership, the ASCC attracted women who were concerned about the risk that cancer posed to themselves and to family members into its ranks.

Such participation of women in cancer control reflected broader social trends. For several decades, women had ascended to important positions in social, educational, and health reform groups. Beginning in the 1880s, women learned about the "science of motherhood," which stressed notions of proper nutrition and care for infants.[7] Since 1904, women had joined antituberculosis societies in the "first truly mass health education campaign directed at a single disease."[8] As women turned to cancer control, they brought with them their experiences of working within female networks to distribute medical information to the general public. Women organized medical lectures for women's clubs, helped orchestrate public health campaigns that targeted particular audiences, and headed philanthropy efforts.[9] In addition to joining the society, women recruited new members and facilitated discourse about cancer in popular American culture.

Many Americans did not need reminders about the seriousness of cancer. In 1914 approximately 75,000 Americans died from the disease every year.[10] The experience of caring for a dying cancer patient was permanently fixed in the memories of many friends and family. Caregivers witnessed cancer's devastation firsthand. This first cancer society in the United States did not teach these individuals about the disease's deadly effects but instead convinced them that education offered a means to curing it.

A Brief History of Cancer

As a disease of antiquity, cancer has attracted the attention of scholars, physicians, and healers for millennia. As early as 1500 B.C.E., the Papyrus Ebers referred to cancer and its deadly effect. When Hippocrates (460–377 B.C.E.), the "father of modern medicine," wrote about cancer, he urged practitioners to resist treating the disease. In his prophetic analysis, he cautioned against treatments that might prove more dangerous than the disease itself.[11]

The earliest cancer narratives focused on adults, usually females, with visible and external cancers such as skin, lip, or breast. Physicians frequently described cases involving a woman with breast cancer, in large part because breast cancer had such obvious manifestations. In spite of Hippocrates's advice, patients continued to seek cures, and many physicians experimented with cancer treatments. Patients turned to balms, herbs, cauterization, and other treatments throughout the centuries.[12]

Until the nineteenth century, most healers treating cancer in the United States adhered to the humoral theory of health. A foundation of medicine for hundreds of years, it explained disease as an imbalance of the four humors: blood, phlegm, black bile, and yellow bile. Believing that cancer resulted from an excess of black bile, healers focused on restoring a balance to the bodily fluids. This process might have included bloodletting, potions, or nutritional therapy. By the nineteenth century, however, scientists turned to pathology, bacteriology, and anatomy as alternative explanations for disease and health. These studies transformed medicine and ushered in a new era of modern cancer theory and therapy.

By the mid-nineteenth century, several scientists had turned their attention to "the cell." Johannes Müller (1801–1858), perhaps the most notable of these scientists, studied cellular growth and formation, offering an initial classification system for tumors. As scholars have noted, "Müller's aim in classifying tumors was an eminently practical one. He wanted the physician to be able to distinguish, for purposes of treatment and prognosis, 'benign' (gutartige) tumors from 'malignant' (bosartige) tumors."[13] Concurrently, the discovery of ether for anesthesia and the advancement of Joseph Lister's theories about aseptic surgery allowed for more careful and safer surgeries. The synthesis of cellular theory, anesthesia for surgery, and aseptic (and later antiseptic) practices created a new era for cancer studies, whereby prognosis was more accurate and hopes for cancer cures were greater.[14]

As physicians increasingly turned to local and aggressive surgery as a cancer treatment, they directed their attention to breast cancer. Johns Hopkins University surgeon William Stewart Halsted gained prominence in the late nineteenth century when he advanced extensive surgical excision for breast tumors. As historian James Olson describes Halsted, "He was the best surgeon in the world, perhaps the best ever. William Stewart Halsted presided over the Johns Hopkins University surgical staff like a medieval prince, dominating those around him by virtue of intellect, technical skill, and scientific judgment."[15] Educated at Andover, Yale, and New York College of Physicians and Surgeons and trained in several European hospitals, Halsted joined Johns Hopkins in 1888. By then, he had already begun practicing radical mastectomies to treat breast cancer, and he continued this practice in the United States. In 1894 he published an influential article, "The Results of Operations for the Cure of Cancer of the Breast," wherein he argued that his clinical experiences with extensive/radical surgery yielded definitive results: patients who were treated with extensive mastectomy lived longer. Halsted and many others believed that cancer began as a local growth and then spread outward. This theory, dominant for much of the twentieth century, would for decades justify radical and often mutilating cancer surgeries.[16]

As a surgeon at Johns Hopkins University, Halsted trained students who conveyed his ideas and practices far and wide. His surgical skills, extensive training, and noteworthy data earned him an international reputation.[17] In order to facilitate successful surgeries, Halsted insisted on germ-free environments during surgery, introduced rubber gloves to the operating room, and initiated surgical residency programs as a way to better train students. He became a disciple of radical surgery during his training in Vienna, Leipzig, and Berlin.

Surgeon Theodor Billroth and cellular pathologist Rudolf Virchow trained him, and Halsted credited German techniques as the basis for his "complete method." To be sure, Halsted's late nineteenth-century studies included many patients who presented with advanced breast cancers. Instead of viewing such cases as hopeless, Halsted believed that his mastectomy procedure could save some lives. As he continued his studies, he became an ardent proponent of early detection as well, believing that survival rates increased when cancer patients presented at earlier stages of the disease. Halsted thus outlined the medical discourse for breast cancer that became dominant in the twentieth century, including an emphasis on lymphatic involvement, stages of disease, and early detection as a way to improve outcomes.[18]

As a distinct field of cancer science emerged, more and more physicians treated the disease.[19] Many physicians believed that the efficacy of surgical treatment would improve if treatment began at the early stages of illness.[20] These physicians wanted patients to gain a keener appreciation of early detection.

Their emphasis on early detection allowed for the creation of public health messages about cancer in the early twentieth century. Physicians pondered ways they might convince the public to consult medical specialists with concerns about cancer. Members of the Clinical Congress of Surgeons of North America voted to establish a "cancer campaign committee" in 1912. This committee would "consider methods of educating the public against cancer."[21] One physician wrote, "There is every reason for enlisting the heartiest public support in the now popular warfare against the white plague."[22] Learning from the National Association for the Study and Prevention of Tuberculosis (TBA), founded in 1904, cancer activists realized the impact that public and lay participation could have on disease control. Moreover, the antituberculosis society offered a model of the positive influence that voluntary efforts could have on teaching the public about contemporary health issues.[23] Indeed, the ASCC recognized its predecessor by promising a "widespread campaign of publicity and education similar to that of the National Association for the study and prevention of tuberculosis."[24] Also like the TBA, this first cancer organization would recruit women to convey its public health message, which served both to legitimize the efforts of medical practitioners in the field and teach audiences about cancer.[25]

Cancer assumed a more prominent place in the popular imagination in the early twentieth century as the threat of contagious diseases lessened and Americans lived longer.[26] Concerned about their own mortality and that of their loved ones, early cancer advocates shared goals of educating the public about cancer and encouraging prompt responses to potential cancer indicators.

Organizing to Educate

Before the creation of the ASCC in 1913, physicians had articulated concern for laypersons' awareness of the disease. In particular, many surgeons and gynecologists believed that female patients only visited physicians in the late stages of cancer. Convinced that earlier diagnosis would facilitate surgical cures, these physicians believed that public education programs might induce patients to visit a physician at the first indication of cancer.[27]

Early twentieth-century medical conference proceedings reflect the medical profession's support for a cancer society. Such a society could coordinate a variety of concerns, such as informing patients about cancer symptoms, encouraging them to consult physicians at the earliest indications of a problem, and promoting routine medical examinations. In 1905 surgeons pronounced their support for such a society at the Annual College of Surgeons gathering. Eight years later, at the 1913 American Gynecological Society meeting, Henry Coe remarked in his presidential address, "We are on the eve of new propaganda which will undoubtedly be productive of great good. This society will render a signal service to humanity in initiating popular education, whatever we may decide are the best channels through which to diffuse the information. The point to be impressed upon the laity is that the earlier the diagnosis, the more radical the operation, the better is the prospect of permanent relief."[28]

Soon thereafter, Dr. Clement Cleveland, another physician who supported the creation of a cancer society that would advance a professional project defined by a narrow conception of disease and a strict definition of early detection, invited prominent doctors to his home. His daughter, Elise Mead, also joined the gathering.[29] Cooperating with the M.D.s who met in her father's home, Mead advocated the idea of creating a group whose goals included educating women about cancer.[30]

The attention that Coe, Cleveland, and Mead placed on education was formally revisited a few months later. On May 22, 1913, fifteen men met at the Harvard Club in New York City to flesh out the details of the first American organization dedicated to cancer awareness. The group consisted of ten male medical professionals (four of whom belonged to the American Gynecological Society) and five laymen.[31] The society elected Wall Street banker George C. Clark as its first president, who would serve until 1919.[32] Indeed, all of the ASCC's leadership positions were held by men, and physicians created the dominant discourse surrounding cancer control, which emphasized patient responsibility. The ASCC's articulated goal was to convince audiences of the benefits of early detection. The founding members reasoned that if audiences gained an awareness of cancer symptoms, responded by visiting a physician, and agreed to recommended treatment (primarily surgery), then cancer could be better controlled.[33] The ASCC modeled itself on the National Association for the Study and Prevention of Tuberculosis and urged advocacy and public education.[34] The ASCC also hoped to debunk the myth that cancer was contagious, and like the TBA, it relied on volunteers to organize its educational campaign.[35]

In spite of a modest budget, within one year of its creation the society had published cancer pamphlets, sponsored speeches on cancer awareness, and convinced magazines to publish articles about the disease and participate in this health campaign. As a survey of the *Readers' Guide to Periodical Literature* suggests, magazines and journals published more articles about cancer awareness after the creation of the society. The ASCC's reliance on the printed word is evident in the establishment of its own printing press in New York City. It immediately launched a monthly publication, *Campaign Notes*. As the society explained, it strived "to collect, collate, and disseminate information concerning the symptoms, diagnosis, treatment, and prevention of cancer, to investigate the conditions under which cancer is found and to compile statistics in regard thereto." These public health reminders served multiple purposes. In addition to promoting cancer awareness, they implicitly praised the medical profession, reminding audiences to incorporate preventative exams into routine behavior, and thereby advanced a professional project.[36]

This medically driven philanthropic cancer organization also welcomed women's participation, however. How did women's early involvement in the society influence the discourse about cancer within lay communities and the educational programs? Although they were excluded from the society's traditional leadership positions, women organized cancer meetings. Often locating these meetings in all-female spaces, women ASCC volunteers contributed to the powerful images of cancer as both a dreaded disease of particular concern to women and a disease that could be controlled by the medical profession. They introduced conversations that demystified cancer and encouraged female audiences to confront it.

In many ways, Elise Mead, a founding member of the ASCC, epitomized the early contribution of women's time and energy. Her interest in the society, evident since her attendance at the 1913 meeting at her father's home, grew into a conviction that public education offered the best means to control cancer. Soon after the ASCC's creation, Mead, as the chair of the temporary Ways and Means Committee, organized a membership drive and regularly tapped into the network of women who might donate to the cause. She proposed various levels of membership in the ASCC, ranging from $5 to $1,000. In 1915, when the society was in financial straits, she solicited fifteen donations of $1,000 to keep the organization financially solvent. Over the next two decades Mead would chair the ASCC Finance Committee, encourage wealthy New York philanthropists to support the organization, and sponsor regular events that directed publicity to cancer.[37]

Influenced by decades of female reform efforts, middle- and upper-class white women, such as Mead, recognized cancer control as a special concern to women. Cancer awareness fit within a social framework that legitimized women's contributions to social reform and public health efforts. Moreover, these women cooperated with male physicians and served the medical profession. Women adopted medical doctrine without critique, reified physicians' already prominent positions, and validated medical theories as useful facts that would lead to increased cancer control in the United States. Mead promulgated such notions while also playing an influential role in the recruitment of early laymen members of the ASCC, including Thomas M. Debevoise, George C. Clark, Thomas Lamont, V. Everit Macy, and John E. Parsons.[38]

From the beginning, then, women secured financial support for the organization and promised to deliver the ASCC message of early detection. Friends and associates of Elise Mead, including Susan Wood, Ella Rigney, and Gertrude Clark, contributed to the society by organizing events that attracted public attention to the cancer problem.[39] Local in scope and organized for a privileged and elite audience of white women, their campaigns introduced cancer philanthropy to New Yorkers. These women repeated medical doctrine with conviction and insisted that cancer could be controlled with popular education campaigns and prompt medical treatment. Journalists shared the excitement of cancer educators and envisioned an end to cancer in the near future. As a writer for *Harper's Weekly* noted in 1913, "a new day is about to dawn."[40]

Some of these women who committed themselves to cancer philanthropy shared their interest with a male relative, as Elise Mead did with her father. Ella Rigney, another influential cancer activist, was the daughter of Frederick Hoffman. Hoffman, a founding member of the ASCC, a statistician for Metropolitan Life, and the author of several articles on cancer control, played a key role in this early movement. In addition, Rigney's husband, Francis Rigney, an illustrator, designed early ASCC posters. Mrs. Rigney started working on cancer control in 1926 and continued her efforts through midcentury, creating such ideas as the little red door campaign.[41]

Women contributed time, energy, and money to promoting the society from the beginning. A glance at the second page of the 1914 *Facts about Cancer* brochure makes this clear. Although no individual men were mentioned, thirteen "philanthropic women" were recognized for their contributions. Among them were such wealthy and notable New Yorkers as Mrs. Frederick W. Vanderbilt, Mrs. John D. Rockefeller Jr., Mrs. Russell Sage, Mrs. James Speyer, Mrs. H. Winthrop Grey, Mrs. John E. Parsons, Mrs. Samuel A. Clark, Mrs. Robert G. Mead, Mrs. Thomas W. Lamont, Mrs. Otto Kahn, Mrs. Morris Jessup, and Mrs. Anson Phelps Stokes. By crediting women in such a public manner, the society endorsed, legitimized, and welcomed women's support.[42]

With their extraordinary financial status, these women represented some of the wealthiest in the United States. Sharing an affinity for philanthropy, they also provided the ASCC with social cachet that drew publicity. Many of these women had a history of donating money in support of social causes, often directing funds to women-centered reform efforts. A few short biographical sketches illustrate this point.

Louise (Mrs. Frederick W.) Vanderbilt earned a reputation in Hyde Park, New York, for her benevolence. She funded youth activities in the neighborhood and offered clothing and toys to those in financial need, especially during the Christmas season. In 1911 she brought the Red Cross movement to Hyde Park and helped establish a District Health Nurse Service in 1917. Her early support of the cancer society reflected both her association with other wealthy women who agreed to support the cause and her dedication to programs meant to improve society and address health concerns.[43]

Abby Aldrich Rockefeller married John D. Rockefeller Jr., the heir to the Standard Oil Company, in 1901. Living in New York City, Mrs. Rockefeller joined Mrs. Vanderbilt in bringing name recognition to the newly created ASCC. She also identified cancer control as a worthwhile cause that complemented many of her charitable and philanthropic tendencies, which included contributions to the American Red Cross, the Young Women's Christian Association, housing programs, art museums, and church clubs.[44]

Mrs. Russell Sage, or Margaret Olivia Slocum Sage, also wielded a remarkable amount of wealth and social prestige. The second wife of a widower, financier, and millionaire who did not believe in charity for the less fortunate, Mrs. Sage nevertheless encouraged philanthropy in subtle ways until his death in 1907. After his death she created the Russell Sage Foundation to promote social betterment. Long affiliated with organized charitable giving and wealthy women's support of it, Mrs. Sage lent her support to the emerging ASCC. Although she would die in 1918, Mrs. Sage lent her prominence and social distinction to the fledgling organization.[45]

Three other women on this list had close personal ties to the ASCC: Ellin Prince Speyer, Mrs. John Parsons, and Gertrude Clark were the spouses of three of the five lay founders of the ASCC. Joining their husbands as supporters of the ASCC, these women offered a female and public face to the society as it articulated its goals of educating the public about cancer and promoting early treatment of the disease. Indeed, by capturing the attention of news organizations, society pages, and other health organizations, the endorsement of such prominent women was crucial to the society's success.

Women also composed the vast majority of the cancer volunteers who distributed awareness literature, staffed information booths at health fairs and in public, and hosted society events. Women embraced education as a way to circulate the message of early detection for breast and reproductive cancers. As volunteers, they spread this message to broader female audiences, encouraging them to care about their cancer risk.

Physicians reinforced the importance of targeting women in cancer education. Dr. Joseph Colt Bloodgood, a student of William Halsted's and one of the most popular cancer specialists of the era, stated emphatically, "Our message to women should be: If you feel, or think you feel, a lump in the breast, or if you notice the slightest irritation of the nipple, see your medical advisor at once." A founding member of the ASCC and reputable cancer specialist from Johns Hopkins University, Bloodgood devoted much of his career to studying breast and cervical cancer. Throughout the 1920s and early 1930s, he continually expressed his belief that cancer awareness/early detection could have a great impact on the cure rates of female cancers. He privileged the wisdom of medical professionals: "The correct message of the medical profession either has not reached the women of America, or, if it has been received, false modesty or some other factor may explain the delay." This sentiment reverberated through his many lectures, which urged self-recognition of female cancer symptoms and subsequent prompt visits to the physician.[46]

Other physicians such as Dr. William Stone shared Bloodgood's assessment. Stone explained, "A special campaign at the same time, all over the country, directed to women for the purpose of acquainting them with the actual facts about uterine cancer, cannot help but materially and immediately reduce the mortality from the disease." He also suggested that women could more effectively spread the mantra of early detection to men and children. Referring to explicit efforts to recruit more women into cancer education work, he wrote, "It appears to be the most fertile field for our educational work, and why not make it, for a time, the chief field of our endeavors?"[47]

Medical professionals thus encouraged women's involvement in early twentieth-century cancer education. Because women did not challenge medical doctrine, but rather adopted the language of conventional medical lessons, they did not threaten the authority of the male doctors. Although women may have tailored the message to better suit a female audience, they did not dispute the doctors' "cancer facts." Nevertheless, by co-opting the messages created by male medical authorities, women entered the realm of medical expertise, albeit in a peripheral and deferential way.

Popular Periodicals and Early Cancer Education Initiatives

Mass publications offered a cost-effective way for cancer educators to reach large audiences of women. Educators encouraged magazines to reprint the ASCC's basic facts about cancer. In addition to these short "factual pieces," they seemed to encourage fictional narratives that combined personal drama with medical theories about cancer. A number of magazines responded to the education initiative. Whereas prior to 1913, articles rarely focused on a specific type of cancer, and none emphasized the particular concerns that women might have about cancer, after the creation of the ASCC, articles implicitly endorsed cancer awareness and frequently alluded to progress in controlling the disease.[48]

By reinforcing the emerging faith in early detection and medical treatment, many of these popular articles also fostered a sense of hope about the disease. Articles such as "What Everyone Should Know about Cancer," "Prevention and Cure of Cancer," and "How Cancer May Be Prevented," encouraged audiences to proactively approach cancer by familiarizing themselves with common symptoms. Others, such as "Surgeons Discuss Cancer Campaign," explicitly recognized the collaborative impulse between the medical profession and the volunteer cancer educators.[49]

Similar patterns held for magazines devoted exclusively to women, including *Good Housekeeping, Ladies' Home Journal*, and *Women's Home Companion*, which published approximately nine articles on cancer between 1900 and 1930. After the creation of the ASCC, the narratives addressed issues of diagnosis, detection, and treatment. Frequently, these articles depicted the cancer patient as female. In 1913 the widely read *Ladies' Home Journal* published Samuel Hopkins Adams's "What Can We Do about Cancer," one of the earliest popular articles to emphasize the merits of cancer control.[50] *Good Housekeeping* subsequently published three similar articles on women and cancer.

After 1913, two distinct themes resonated in popular periodicals: emphasis on the warning signs of cancer and attention to the value

FIGURE 1. Cancer Articles in Popular Magazines

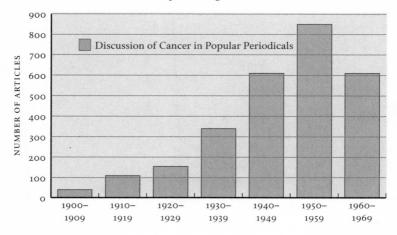

of early cancer treatment. Many articles listed the ASCC's seven major warning signs of cancer:

1. Unusual fatigue and weakness
2. A lump in the breast
3. Irregular vaginal bleeding or discharge
4. Sores that won't heal
5. Persistent indigestion
6. A mole that changes in appearance
7. Unusual bowel movements

Notably, this list, prominently displayed on most ASCC publications and posters and featured in popular periodicals, spoke specifically to female audiences in the second and third warning signs. Without overwhelming readers with fear about this potentially fatal disease, articles attempted to explain the behavior of cancer. Endorsing theories of local growth, these articles encouraged patients to consult physicians at the earliest indication of abnormality (for example, an unusual breast growth or vaginal discharge) so that surgeons could excise the tumor. Again, emphasizing the importance of early detection, articles in popular magazines implied that early surgical inter-

FIGURE 2. Popular Periodicals Discuss Women and Cancer

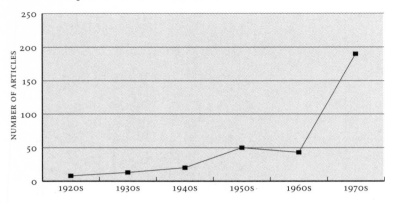

vention could cure cancer, or at least significantly decrease the number of women dying from cancer.[51] As one example, "What Can We Do about Cancer?"—the 1913 article in *Ladies' Home Journal*—included the opinions of various medical specialists. Most of the interviewed subjects admitted there was no known cause of cancer but advised readers to "educate the people to save themselves."[52] When reading such articles, many women learned to trust physicians and defer to their treatment protocol, prioritizing scientific knowledge in modern society.

Articles in women's magazines also focused on women's experiences with the disease. Authors often introduced generic ideas pertinent to all cancers but then focused on the diagnosis and treatment of breast and reproductive cancer. For example, in a section of "What Can We Do about Cancer" that was dedicated specifically to cancers common in women, author Samuel Hopkins Adams explained the need to remove the entire breast if cancer was diagnosed. For uterine cancer, Adams insisted that early diagnosis would dramatically change one's chance of survival and again emphasized the value of a "radical operation."[53]

In 1922 Dr. Harvey Wiley, the director of the *Good Housekeeping* Bureau of Foods, Sanitation, and Health, wrote an article for the magazine entitled, "*If* You *Think* You Have *a Cancer*." He explained,

"The female is much more subject to cancer than the male after the age of maturity is reached. The mammary glands and the uterus, with its appendages are the two vulnerable points in women particularly attractive to cancer."[54] Another article in *Good Housekeeping* by Dr. Joseph Colt Bloodgood focused more specifically on cervical cancer. Bloodgood relished the opportunity to address the female readership: "False modesty, chiefly on the part of the public press, has made it difficult to get the correct information to the public."[55] More specialized women's magazines, such as *Woman Citizen*, asked, "Must Women Die of Cancer?"[56]

In the early decades of the twentieth century, women's magazines directed equal attention to various types of female cancers, or those cancers specific to women. For instance, many articles referred to the risk of breast cancer while also highlighting the dangers of "reproductive cancers." (Popular conversations of cancer lumped specific reproductive cancers together into a single category.) However, in the first part of the twentieth century, this category of "reproductive cancers" posed a greater risk for women than any other type of cancer. By midcentury, however, with the advent of the Pap smear, mortality rates from cervical cancer began to decline steadily. After the feminist health movement, Betty Ford's and Happy Rockefeller's diagnosis, and the availability of mammography, breast cancer received exponentially greater attention, as shown in figure 3.[57]

Less obvious than the trend for women's magazines to focus on female cancers, many articles in general magazines also zeroed in on women's experiences. Although an article's title might suggest a broad survey of cancer knowledge, the piece would frequently present a detailed discussion of women and cancer. For example, in *Harper's Weekly* one journalist's discussion of "How Cancer May Be Prevented" focused so much attention on women and cancer that a reader might perceive cancer as an exclusively female problem. As the article concluded, "This is the news to be disseminated throughout the length and breadth of the land: to be carried to every mother, wife, and sister."[58]

The focus on female audiences, and to a lesser extent on female cancers, framed popular perceptions of cancer in the 1910s through the 1930s. Cancer was commonly portrayed as a women's issue. The emerging public discourse about cancer fostered public awareness that women should be particularly vigilant about cancer care.

In 1923 *Hygeia*, a magazine committed to bridging the ideas of the medical profession and the general public, began monthly publication. Often found in the waiting rooms of physicians' offices and sponsored by the American Medical Association, the journal offered medical theory without jargon and targeted a nonprofessional audience. More important, it stressed practical measures a reader might take to maintain or improve her or his health. Its range of subjects indicated an audience of both men and women; however, a disproportionate number of articles seemed to address female readers. *Hygeia* epitomized an increasingly evident twentieth-century trend—the blurring of boundaries between medical and popular literature and between a professional and lay audience. It frequently discussed the medical definitions of cancer, making this a more accessible topic for the public in general, and women in particular.

For example, in 1931 *Hygeia* published "Facing Cancer with Courage." The byline identified the author as "One Who Has Tried It and Achieved Success." An image of a serious, presumably worried woman accompanied the text. This article not only encouraged the reader to learn about cancer but also offered advice about dealing with the psychological aspects of cancer: "It is a wise thing to look the word cancer straight in the face so that the sight of it in print may not send a shiver through you. Then read the literature about it—not the hysterical literature of the quacks, who alas, still flourish, but the sane, scientific articles that appear frequently in the magazines and the bulletins that are issued by research organizations."[59]

Perhaps as a way to facilitate this courageous, "look cancer straight in the face" attitude, ASCC literature and popular periodicals correctly informed women that the majority of lumps in the breast were noncancerous or benign. Articles adamantly stressed the need for a professional opinion in determining the nature of a lump, routinely reinforcing the idea that the medical profession could cure cancer

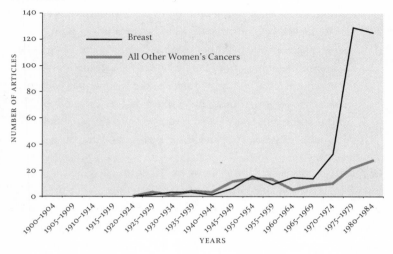

when patients followed instructions.[60] Science ascended as the tool for diagnosis, outstripping all other forms of knowledge.[61]

With the authority of science behind them, these early articles set in motion the idea that women bore responsibility in cancer diagnosis. Many insisted that women could and should recognize suspicious growths. As cancer, and the cancer patient, became gendered female, medical messages increasingly blamed women and implied that they assumed some culpability for a later stage diagnosis. By focusing on the female patient's responsibility to detect cancer promptly, health messages conveyed by female volunteers and the ASCC served to chastise female cancer patients and alleviate any responsibility that physicians bore for poor medical outcomes. Although the messages were conveyed by female volunteers, the strict adherence to male medical expertise silenced any critique of cancer control.

In 1926, *Hygeia* published an article that trivialized women's fear of cancer and that again directed the focus of cancer control to patients' ignoring the limitations of science:

It has been concluded that when a woman discovers a lump in her breast she feels it perhaps a half a dozen times and then asks the opinion of her mother, who likewise feels it two or three times to be certain it is a lump; then she consults neighbors and friends, who, after considerable manipulation, tell her what she already knew in the first place, that it is a lump. . . . If a woman has a lump in her breast she should understand that to feel it once is all-sufficient. Her next step should be to go to the best possible physician . . . and abide by his decision.[62]

This excerpt epitomizes the issues of blame outlined above, but it also exposes the complexity inherent to any discussion about the public' and private dimensions of cancer. Although the article rebuked a woman for delaying her treatment, it also acknowledged her numerous conversations with other women in her community. According to this author, a woman might talk with her mother and female friends before consulting a physician. Moreover, she would ask other women to feel her suspicious growth. Although the article both dismissed and undermined the importance of the network of women who shared concerns about their health, it recognized the importance of this community in women's lives. As this article suggests, the cancer education movement at first weakened, and may have undermined, the knowledge produced when women turned to each other for advice. Instead, it encouraged women to consult medical authority. The ASCC and its corps of volunteers privileged scientific knowledge and openly criticized the parochial nature of women's knowledge that might postpone a visit to the physician.

Such patronizing themes implying that female cancer victims were at fault for their failure to respond to symptoms routinely appeared in a variety of popular magazines. As one journalist stated, "The worst possible course to pursue is to wait to see what will happen before seeking a medical opinion. If cancer is present it should receive treatment at once. Untreated cancer invariably causes death. Any delay in starting treatment may result in the cancer spreading too far to be cured by any form of treatment."[63] Certainly, these articles meant to encourage early detection, yet they failed to address the web of reasons that women may have resisted consulting a physician. By focusing on women's naiveté, however, the ASCC and its advocates could maintain their devotion to early detection, while ignoring the dearth of epidemiological studies to support this theory.[64]

Consequently, popular advice frequently echoed patriarchal and elitist notions about women's position in a male-dominated medical profession. As one journal described, "Nodules which may be early cancer of the breast can be easily detected by any woman who is intelligent and enlightened enough to adopt the habit of periodically examining her own breast tissue. The word 'enlightened' in this instance has a very important connotation. It refers to the unfortunate prudishness which makes some women loathe to take an intelligent and impersonal interest in the well-being of their own bodies."[65] These references to "unfortunate prudishness" or false modesty dismissed the ubiquitous barriers to women's health care throughout the United States. For many, the cost of visiting a doctor for a mere suspicion of cancer proved prohibitive. For others, racism operated to exclude women of color from accessible health care. Geographic isolation prevented many women from visiting a doctor for non-emergencies. Still others negotiated their cancer suspicions in individual and contemplative ways that included consultation with friends, relatives, or alternative healers before visiting a physician. The quotation above captures the condescension in medical discourse, which treated women's behavior as immature and unenlightened while reiterating the value of scientific knowledge.

The reference to prudishness also highlights a key variability in the early awareness campaigns. When journals published anecdotal evidence about women who hesitated to consult physicians, the importance of early detection was reinforced, but so, too, was the message of blaming the patient. If and when the discourse about cancer portrayed the female patient as noncompliant and therefore culpable, it exonerated the medical profession.

By the end of the 1930s, many readers had learned to detect cancer symptoms in their own bodies and knew of the individual responsibility that they had to assume when confronting cancer. As the education message stressed, "Be watchful of yourself, without undue worry." (Most articles especially encouraged women over the age of thirty-five, who faced a higher risk of cancer, to be vigilant.)[66] In addition, writers encouraged readers to recognize cancer symptoms in friends, relatives, and neighbors. One journalist explained, "I sincerely trust that every one who reads these words will use his best endeavors to send cancer patients to hospitals at the earliest possible moment."[67]

As the twentieth century progressed, early detection messages that targeted female audiences gradually began to offer more specific advice about ways that women might identify cancer. Vague recommendations that encouraged self-examination of breasts became more detailed, perhaps creating a precursor for the modern breast self-examination. Moreover, cancer awareness advocates, journalists, and volunteers who were committed to educating women about breast and uterine cancer encouraged public discussion of the disease. Yet some issues remained absent from public discourse, including the discomfort a woman might feel in a predominantly male medical profession, the effects of mastectomy, and the stigma some people attached to a disease in private body parts. Breasts symbolized women's sexuality and femininity, and public discussion of breasts, no matter what the context, usually took the sensitivity of the subject into account. As a result, educators frequently relied on innuendos. For instance, a woman might notice a lump while showering or if her hand "brushed against her breast" while dressing. As one woman explained, "Standing under the shower that night I noticed for the first time a lump on my breast. It wasn't a large one. It wasn't any bigger than the tip of my finger." Discussions of reproductive cancers emphasized irregular vaginal discharges and the need to consult a physician, rarely describing the appearance, thickness, or frequency of irregular discharge.[68]

In the 1940s even more magazines published articles on cancer. Part of this shift can be explained by World War II and the renewed interest in medicine, science, and technology that accompanied it.[69]

However, the midcentury increase in the number of magazines that were aimed at female audiences may have been an equally influential factor. Beginning in 1939 and evident for the next two decades, many magazines redefined their readership by embracing an exclusively female audience. *Glamour, Seventeen, Redbook, Cosmopolitan,* and *Mademoiselle* were transformed into "women's magazines" that addressed issues of concern for a female readership. For decades, cancer educators had been casting cancer as a special concern for women. Now they had a greater number of popular periodicals that served this audience.[70] As a result, more articles, whose cancer discussions were informed by the ASCC and its goals, identified the different types of cancer, cancers particular to women or "female cancers," the potential impact of early detection, and the insistent message that prompt treatment cured cancer.

Other Cancer Education Programs

ASCC efforts to educate the public went beyond popular magazines. Cancer awareness volunteers worked inventively to expand audiences and increase public consciousness of cancer. As the ASCC explained, "The means employed in giving out the available information comprise practically all the methods known to public health agencies and include lectures, newspaper and magazine articles, moving pictures, radio talks, posters, circulars, handbooks, a periodical and private correspondence."[71] The ASCC convinced high schools and health fairs to include information about cancer. Women in the ASCC made liaisons with faculty and public health advocates, working vigorously to spread the message of early detection. "Into America's schools and homes will go the word that cancer in its early stages is curable," advocates cheered.[72] These daily acts of education, frequently performed by women, sustained the message that early detection offered the best means to control cancer and fostered optimism about its cure. In 1921 the ASCC began sponsoring an annual "cancer week," during which newspapers printed a series of articles on cancer, radio programs included informative spots on the disease, and the ASCC displayed posters on street corners, on billboards, and in trolley cars. The ASCC "conservatively estimated" that 10 million people learned about cancer in its first annual cancer week.[73]

The ASCC also cooperated with the observances of National Negro Health Week. This annual program, begun in 1915, urged audiences to "help yourself and your community to better health."[74] In 1925, when program organizers set aside one day per week for a specific topic, they identified cancer as a key concern of the African American health movement. The educational aims of the ASCC aligned nicely with the goals of National Negro Health Week. As one newspaper headline reported, "Colored Organizations to Cooperate with Authorities in Education Drive." The ASCC readily shared its promotional literature that encouraged audiences to learn about cancer, its symptoms, and the importance of physician consultation but said nothing about the neglect of health-care issues for African Americans or how this neglect affected cancer diagnosis and treatment.[75]

Additional efforts to teach the public about cancer included increased cooperation between radio networks and cancer educators. By the mid-1930s, the educational campaign could increasingly be heard on the airwaves: "In the process of developing various methods of reaching the lay public in the campaign of cancer education the radio has begun to assume a position of outstanding importance."[76]

Although popular periodicals, radio shows, and classroom lectures reached millions of readers and listeners, film offered visual stories of cancer that complemented the other narratives. This alternative form of cancer education first appeared in 1920. Early cancer education films exposed emerging paradigms in cancer awareness that gendered patients and physicians, reinforced developing discourse about cancer hopes and fears, and fostered the creation of public places to talk about cancer.

In 1920 the ASCC produced *The Great Peril*, a black-and-white, fifteen-minute silent film that follows the life of Gordon Crane, a young doctor devoted to cancer research. His passion for work includes his quest to inform the public that "this disease is the greatest menace

the world has ever known." The plot revolves around Gordon's relationship to Margaret, his fiancée, and their efforts to balance their
devotion to each other with Gordon's long work hours. The opening
scene features Gordon sitting at his desk, writing a book on "the great
peril." His father, also a doctor, enters the office to remind Gordon
that he must balance his cancer research and his medical practice.
This early reminder about Gordon's professional responsibilities reflected the historical reality that men dominated clinical and research
centers for cancer. The character of Gordon Crane thus embodied the
dominant gender ideologies of the era, which portrayed medical authorities as privileged white males.[77]

Margaret, waiting outside Gordon's office, joins him as he leaves
for a meeting. The viewer learns that Gordon gives speeches throughout town, spreading the message of early cancer detection. The camera pans his middle-class audience, first focusing on a group of four
listeners, consisting of three middle-aged white women and one
white man. The camera then focuses on one woman who stares with
intense concentration. This film, like much cancer awareness literature, thus identified women as the primary audience for cancer
awareness. Very often, women were portrayed as apprehensive but
intensely curious about this disease. Also typical of cancer films, men
were most often portrayed as the all-knowing doctors.

Dr. Crane's lecture includes three main points, all printed as text
in between moving images. First, Gordon emphasizes, "The public
must understand that cancer can be cured if treated early." He then
explains that cancer was not a germ, and it was neither contagious
nor hereditary. Finally, Gordon warns against alternative cures and
remedies, reminding viewers that professional doctors offered the
best treatment for cancer.

Meanwhile, in a subplot, Margaret meets with her mother, who looks
weary. Despite Margaret's insistence that her mother should visit a
doctor, her mother refuses. Gordon continues his work, constantly
reminding the viewer that cancer could be cured if, and only if, it was
detected early. Predictably, Margaret's mother continues to worsen.

In the final scene of the short film, Gordon examines Margaret's mother. He diagnoses her with advanced cancer and explains that he cannot help her. Of course, if she had visited him at the first sign of the disease, he might have been able to cure it. As the film nears its end, Gordon remains the hero, while both women assume some blame for this late-stage cancer diagnosis. The daughter has failed to convince her mother to visit a doctor sooner, and her mother has ignored the dire nature of her condition. Despite Margaret's sadness about her mother's condition, Margaret now recognizes the importance of Gordon's work. The course of events reassures her that she wants to marry Gordon.

This early ASCC film reflected a tendency to exaggerate both the obvious nature of cancer symptoms and patients' tendencies to delay. At the same time, it normalized physicians' ability to cure. It also epitomized gendered assumptions about medicine and professionalism, where men acted as dominant authorities and women were depicted as passive audiences.

Clearly, the film's principal message stressed the value of early detection. However, a subtler message implied that if a woman died from cancer, she should assume some blame. The mother's refusal to seek early medical care led to her death. The primary culprit was not the disease, or the doctor unable to treat it, but the patient. By featuring a female victim, the film, and cancer education campaigns in general, represented the fact that more women died from the disease than men did; yet, these messages also stigmatized the cancer victim. The positions women assumed (as audience members or educators) increased their access to knowledge but, at the same time, limited their agency by portraying their dependency on (typically male) physicians.

As another example of the functioning of gender ideology in this film, the second female character, Margaret, played the role of a dutiful and supportive fiancée who recognized the importance of her husband's career. Although her character remained undeveloped, by the film's end she assumed the "supportive" role that women were meant to play in both their personal relationships and in their alliance with the medical profession and its commitment to early detection.

Upon second reading, the film depicts a more complicated rendition of the reality of cancer and gender roles in the early twentieth century. Women in this film, as both audience members and educators, participated in a conversation about their bodies. The featured seminar offered women scientific/professional knowledge and allowed them to claim it and spread it to a broader audience of women. In this, the film recognized the important role of women in public health campaigns. Although it acknowledged the (masculine) authority of science and medicine, it captured the experience of women who discussed cancer within a female community before they consulted a male medical professional. Women's confidence in one another was undermined in this film, and viewers were meant to disregard this knowledge in favor of science. The inclusion of this aspect of women's experience nevertheless suggests the pervasiveness of female networks of care in the early twentieth century and the concerted effort to disrupt these networks in favor of medical authority.

Moreover, although it is obscured by Gordon Crane, who is presented as the dominant authority, the influential role of female cancer educators and organizers can be inferred from this film. The film ignored any details that would reveal who organized the meeting, invited the audience, or coordinated with the physician-speaker. It is nonetheless likely that female volunteers arranged such meetings.

Although *The Great Peril* underscored the value of early detection, early detection had obvious limitations for cancer care. Namely, surgery as a cure only applied to those cancers with "early manifestations" or noticeable symptoms. These included external cancers, such as cancer of the skin, the lip, and the breast. They also included some internal cancers, such as cervical or uterine cancer, that exhibited early indications of the disease—in this case, irregular vaginal discharge or bleeding. Despite these limitations, the film worked to spread the message of early detection, which was perhaps the only proactive measure the ASCC could take to reduce cancer mortality in the first decades of the twentieth century.

Expanding the Campaign

The ASCC celebrated its early achievements, including the distribution of this educational film, in its 1925 publication, *The American Society for the Control of Cancer: Its Objects and Methods and Some of the Visible Results of Its Work*. The society highlighted its educational achievements while insisting that it had even more potential: "The commission believes that this report proves conclusively that cancer education pays, and should be continued by all proper means, and with increased vigor under the stimulating influence of success." It employed statistics to validate its work. Very often, the ASCC tracked progress in its education programs for women by emphasizing the decreased time span between initial breast and cervical cancer symptoms and doctor consultations. Pamphlets also described case studies of breast and uterine cancer and suggested that the increase in breast exams in the 1920s was a direct result of the ASCC education campaign.[78]

Meanwhile, the ASCC continued to publish educational pamphlets. In 1931 *Important Facts for Women about Tumors* explained, "This pamphlet presents the more important facts about tumors which are of special concern to women, including information as to their nature, their symptoms, their prevention, and their cure." Clearly, women remained a target audience for cancer education. The booklet focused on breast and uterine cancer and emphasized the potential for early detection of these cancers.[79] The society now also sought to expand its audience by reproducing its pamphlet in several languages for immigrant communities in the United States and for international distribution.[80]

The content and language in this pamphlet reflected both the breadth and limits of a public discussion about female cancers in 1931, and the shifts that had occurred since 1913. This pamphlet spoke freely about the female body and abnormal growths in the breast and uterus. Typical of cancer literature in this era, it still stressed the importance of early detection but also stated that "dangerous varieties of these tumors present such apparently trivial symptoms in their beginning that the patient often does not appreciate their true nature and so disregards the early warning."[81] The pamphlet did not admonish patients for having ignored cancer symptoms; rather, it informed women of the early symptoms of cancer and reminded readers that "among all the tumors in the human body there are none which yield more readily to early treatment than those which are peculiar to women."[82] Then, and for many decades to follow, many physicians perceived the early stages of female cancers to be entirely local and surgically accessible. This assumption reinforced the emphasis that cancer awareness programs placed on women and early detection.

One section of the pamphlet, entitled "Tumors of the Breast," presented a summary of breast cancer. First, it offered a blunt explanation of breast cancer indicators, including unusual lumps in the breast, bleeding nipples, and a wide variety of tumors. Second, it emphasized that physical examinations should be conducted by medical professionals, who were still almost exclusively male during this era. (Although it suggested that physical exams might indicate breast cancer, it emphasized that only a surgical biopsy could confirm that diagnosis.) Although the pamphlet reflected a more open discussion of the breast cancer and other cancer symptoms, information about treatment remained elusive. The pamphlet vaguely mentioned surgery as a cure for breast cancer but said nothing specific about mastectomy, then the primary surgical treatment for any breast cancer diagnosis. Finally, while the pamphlet reminded the reader that diagnosis at an "early stage" was critical, it offered a limited description of the medical distinctions between different stages of the disease, a concept that was still unclear in much popular and medical literature in the first half of the twentieth century.

Likewise, another section, "Tumors of the Uterus," described symptoms of uterine cancer in a straightforward manner: "This [unusual discharge] may appear between the menstrual periods as a simple 'spotting' or slight staining following a bowel movement, sexual intercourse, the use of a douche, or some exertion."[83] Again, the pamphlet failed to describe the surgical treatment that followed a cancer diagnosis. The pamphlet made frequent reference to an "internal pelvic exam," but it did not describe who performed the exam, the steps it involved, or what the procedure included. Reflecting the optimism that surrounded cancer education, the pamphlet suggested, "Cancer of the uterus is curable, if recognized and treated early; it is fatal when neglected." Finally, the pamphlet explained, "To postpone such consultation with a physician because of a dread that cancer may be discovered is the height of imprudence."[84] Whereas other publications would suggest that women postponed treatment due to "false modesty," this publication suggested that a real fear of the diagnosis deterred many women from seeking early medical consultation. The pamphlet included rhetoric now common to the cancer education crusade. Visit a doctor regularly, insist that a physician examine any suspicious growths, and confront the medical costs. (The authors insisted that any "competent medical service" would honor all patients regardless of financial status.)[85]

By the 1930s, American concern for cancer was evident in the global arena as well. In 1926 the ASCC sponsored the first international conference. It invited speakers from Europe to meet in New York at the Mohonk Cancer Symposium "for the purpose of considering the prevention and cure of cancer from a practical standpoint." Over one hundred medical personnel attended, sixteen as representatives from overseas. They compared organized cancer control movements in the United States, England, France, Switzerland, Belgium, Italy, and Germany; methods of detection and treatment; and mortality rates. Papers that focused on cancer control in the United States reviewed the accomplishments of the ASCC and offered direction for the organization's future. The concern for women and cancer was evident in these conference proceedings. Several presenters emphasized the need to pay even more attention to women, female cancers, and early detection.[86]

Although the ASCC had accomplished much in the 1910s and 1920s, it took decades for the message of early detection to become part of mainstream culture. Many of the cancer awareness events were limited to the East Coast, and most volunteers derived from a privileged segment of the U.S. population, primarily middle- and upper-class white women. Rural women and many communities of color still knew little about cancer and lacked access to even basic health-care services.[87]

Despite these limitations, the ASCC had gained recognition and become a national voice and cancer authority within the United States. It continued to reflect the interests of its founding members and leaders—the medical professionals. The ASCC encouraged the public to consult the medical profession regularly. In a 1931 press release it stated, "If people wish the greatest possible protection against cancer and other disease they should, while they are well, select a family physician if they can afford it, or a clinic if they cannot. They should visit that physician or clinic while they are well and should ask not only for an examination but for advice on the rules of health and on the earliest symptoms of disease." This statement garnered attention from newspapers throughout the country, including the *New York Times*, which published it in its Sunday edition. By the early 1930s, when the ASCC issued press releases, it gained the attention of the news media.[88]

The press release not only reiterated the medical consensus on cancer, but it also clearly served the medical profession and its effort to control and regulate standard medical practices in the United States. As a consequence, it served to weaken nonprofessional bonds, such as the informal networks of women, by devaluing nonclinical knowledge. Responding to the rise in alternative cancer therapy, more commonly referred to as medical fraud practiced by "quacks," the ASCC urged audiences to seek out licensed medical professionals and consult them for regular exams.[89]

As the twentieth century progressed, the ASCC rigidly clung to the philosophy of its founding members. It adhered to its doctrine of early detection and promised that surgical treatment offered the best hope for curing cancer.[90] Likewise, popular literature hailed the advancement of surgery but failed to convey details about the process and effects of hysterectomies and radical mastectomies. Cancer activism remained in its infancy in these early decades, but philanthropic women and female volunteers within the ASCC endorsed the messages set forth by physicians and encouraged women to participate in the culture of cancer detection. Together, these women and the ASCC made inroads into incorporating cancer control into American popular culture.

ASCC and the Government

By 1930 women's contributions to cancer control included efforts to publicize cancer and spread the message of early detection to various female networks.[91] In just over two decades, the society had distributed thousands of pamphlets about cancer, produced *The Great Peril*, convinced the government to endorse a national cancer week, and encouraged dozens of magazines, newspapers, and radio stations to teach the public about cancer. Moreover, women invited female audiences to cancer lectures that stressed the importance of recognizing early indications of breast and reproductive cancers.

In the early decades of the twentieth century, however, the federal government remained largely uninterested in the cancer problem. The U.S. Public Health Service assumed some responsibility for the discussion, research, and statistical evaluations of cancer, but the disease was certainly not a priority for elected officials.[92] In fact, other than a few outspoken individual congressional representatives, the disease rarely attracted the attention of politicians before 1937.

In the 1920s Senator Matthew M. Neely of West Virginia, a Democrat and therefore in the minority party, initiated the first extended discussion of cancer in Congress. A politician concerned about cancer, Neely introduced a bill designed to solve the "cancer problem" in February 1927. He proposed that Congress offer a $5 million reward to anyone who could cure cancer. Subsequently, over 2,500 letters arrived, most proposing outrageous cures for cancer.[93] Neely included a sample of these letters in the *Congressional Record*. One person sent Neely an anointed handkerchief with instructions to lay it over the patient "in the name of Jesus"; another suggested a caustic remedy of ten grains of arsenic, one egg white, and soot from a woodstove;

another recommended an herbal drink with boggo, stoneflower, and wild vineyard. As Neely explained, the letters "convinced me that the plan to offer a reward for a cancer cure set forth in my bill was imperfect, if not utterly futile."[94]

The next year Neely tried another approach to the cancer problem. He dramatically introduced the topic of the disease to the Senate with metaphors that emphasized cancer's destructive nature, such as "a monster that is more insatiable than the guillotine." He articulated concern about women who, "because of the unusual susceptibility of the female breast and organs of reproduction," died more frequently from cancer.[95] As he explained, "Medical science has conquered yellow fever, diphtheria, typhoid, and smallpox. Medical science has robbed even leprosy and tuberculosis of their terrors. But in spite of all that physicians, surgeons, biologists, and all other scientists have done, cancer remains the unconquered, the unconquerable, and defiant foe of the human race. It is to-day more menacing and deadly and irresistible than ever before."[96] As Neely noted in his 1928 speech, the government's total cancer appropriations amounted to just $400,000 per year, while Congress appropriated $10 million to eradicate corn borer, $5 million to study tuberculosis and paratuberculosis in animals, and $2 million for meat inspection. Neely's bill to fund further cancer research ultimately gained Senate approval but failed in the House of Representatives. Neely's near success indicated that the government had begun to recognize cancer as a significant public health concern, though it was still unwilling to invest much in this problem.[97]

Individual members of Congress thus expressed occasional interest in cancer; however, throughout the early 1930s most federal representatives ignored the disease, perhaps overwhelmed by the enormity of the problem. As historian James T. Patterson has argued, "The striking aspect of the 1920s and 1930s was the groping, often desperate, quest for a solution to the ever enigmatic problem of cancer."[98] Moreover, unlike the ASCC literature that tended to target women, the government introduced no gender-specific programs.[99]

In the early 1930s, however, the War Department issued a medical recommendation for women that endorsed routine cancer screening. On March 11, 1931, the War Department published Circular No. 25, a three-page document entitled "Annual Physical Examinations of Women."[100] Referring to the army's history of "periodic physical examination as an effective measure in preventative medicine" for enlisted men, this publication advocated regular physical exams for women. Specifically, it stressed, "*The periodic physical examination of the wives of officers and enlisted men offers the best hope for any detection of these conditions* [chronic diseases and degenerative conditions] *at a stage in which they are amenable to cure or amelioration.*"[101]

Such "chronic and degenerative" diseases included cancers, and the directive for "periodic physical examination" introduced routine pelvic exams as part of standard care for women. The circular offered some of the first clear evidence of the government's cooperation in the cancer crusade and its recognition of cancer as a specific concern for women. The circular encouraged medical personnel to "give earnest consideration to the suggestion of establishing an annual physical examination among the adult women." Moreover, it adopted the message promulgated by the ASCC that encouraged dissemination of this knowledge to the masses: "By encouraging periodic examinations through the medium of health talks, suitable publicity in local service publications, distribution of leaflets, and personal advice at gynecological and obstetrical clinics already established, the interest of the women of the Army can be aroused as to the need for guarding themselves against the danger of chronic and degenerative diseases. Once the interest of women in this matter is aroused, it is believed that they can be depended on to carry on educational work themselves along this line."[102]

Additional points contained in the circular emphasized the importance of regular exams, especially after childbirth. The role of nurses in this program was of primary importance because "intimate contact with women of all classes places [a nurse] in a strategic position for advising periodic examinations and for persuading women to apply to physicians." Perhaps with an eye toward male physicians and the personal nature of this exam, the circular also urged women to come in pairs if a nurse could not be present for the examination.[103]

The War Department circular ended with a curious summation: "It should be clearly understood that these examinations are purely voluntary and no coercion whatever should be used. It is believed desirable that no record of such examinations be maintained at the station, but each woman examined should be given a brief confidential memorandum enumerating any defects of importance. She should be advised to preserve this memorandum and present it to the medical officers making subsequent examinations." Encouraging doctors to offer women their medical records might have led to poor record keeping, but it also ensured that women would be aware of their health status and that travel or changes in the physicians on base would not lead to the misplacement of women's health records.[104]

Conclusion

Women who participated in cancer control in the early twentieth century had one goal, and they achieved this within the social structure afforded them. Relying on the founding principle of the ASCC—that early detection offered the best means of controlling cancer—women launched efforts to inform female audiences about the symptoms of breast and reproductive cancers. As one journalist concluded in an article on cancer in women, "The educational campaign against cancer is not conducted to create worry or to startle the public. It is not done to scare you to death, but it is done to frighten you into life."[105]

Since the beginning of the twentieth century, cancer had been a standard subject in medical discourse. Beginning in 1913, it became a common subject for popular discourse as well. With the creation of the ASCC and the grassroots activism of hundreds of women throughout the United States, cancer narratives gradually appeared in popular periodicals, educational films, professional manuals for lay populations, and even within government documents. Adopting the language of preventive medicine, women endorsed the medical doctrine that early detection averted the onset of the most dangerous part of the disease—its advanced and aggressive phase. Female cancer educators introduced a sense of hope and optimism that became a critical component of the ASCC and its mission.

Early detection, however, placed a considerable burden on the patient to recognize early cancer symptoms and to consult medical professionals quickly and regularly. As Frederick Hoffman concluded in his 1925 report *Some Cancer Facts and Fallacies*, "The outstanding fact of my own investigations is the indifference on the part of the cancer patient to the supremely important *time factor* in the progress of the disease."[106] Nevertheless, cancer control in the early twentieth century provided a sense that individuals could manage this disease in cooperation with the medical profession. For women, the campaign recognized their particular vulnerability to cancer. It fostered female networks committed to educating one another about cancer and health while simultaneously advancing a professional project that prioritized scientific knowledge and medical expertise.

2

Expanding Networks of Women
THE AMANDA SIMS MEMORIAL FUND AND
THE WOMEN'S FIELD ARMY

Stories about women with cancer, cancer articles in popular women's magazines, the distribution of pamphlets that listed warning signs for breast and reproductive cancers, and women's involvement in awareness programs and cancer philanthropy all contributed to the notion that cancer was of particular concern to women. Throughout the 1930s women organized themselves, in a more formal manner, to advance cancer awareness. This chapter examines the creation of an "army" of female cancer educators, the involvement of dozens of women's clubs in cancer awareness efforts, and the rise of female networks within American society and culture that promulgated the message of early detection.

Two organizations coordinated women's cancer education initiatives during the 1930s: the Amanda Sims Memorial Fund (ASMF) and the Women's Field Army (WFA). The ASMF was formed in 1930 when Amanda Sims's son made a donation for cancer research in memory of his mother.[1] This donation funded a female-centered cervical cancer education program that targeted mothers in Baltimore and neighboring areas. A few years later, the WFA was formed as an affiliate of the American Society for the Control of Cancer (ASCC). Recognizing women's central role in cancer education, and working to validate the notion that education would decrease cancer mortality, the ASCC recruited women by the thousands to join this organization. Curiously modeled on a traditionally masculine institution, the WFA maintained an exclusively female membership, and the leaders of this organization were some of the most influential clubwomen of the early twentieth century. By employing images of war, the WFA reinforced the notion that women could fight cancer by joining the army of soldiers combating it.[2] Members of the Women's Field Army advanced a female-centered dialogue about cancer awareness and recruited women throughout the nation to participate in its goal of teaching the public about cancer warning signs. In this organization, women also adopted a cancer discourse that viewed cancer as a public health issue.

Women served as "middle figures" in the cancer education movement, which ensured that ideas created by the medical community would reach the lay population.[3] The ASMF and the WFA provided formal structures that encouraged women to participate in the amelioration of medical problems. Although women remained underrepresented as physicians and scientists, health organizations offered women leadership positions in popular education programs.[4] Female volunteers communicated the ideas articulated by the members of the ASCC (primarily male gynecologists, surgeons, and physicians) to a large audience (primarily females, often middle- to upper-class white women). The ASMF and WFA workers sought to demystify cancer by providing women with the knowledge that allowed them to participate more fully in medical experiences, diagnosis, and treatment.

Both of these organizations relied heavily on the extensive networks of women's clubs in the 1930s and shared mutual concerns about women and health in the United States. Each organization educated female audiences about cancer, fostered a sense of female responsibility for health, and encouraged women to demand routine physical examinations for cancer. After the creation of the WFA, the female membership of the ASCC expanded dramatically. Hundreds of thousands of women joined the ASCC in this new initiative that was meant to expand female cancer awareness programs throughout the country.

The Amanda Sims Memorial Fund

In December 1930 John H. Sims, a carpenter from Boomer, West Virginia, sent his U.S. senator, Matthew Neely, a check for $1,000. The donation was made in the memory of his mother, Amanda Sims, who had died of cancer in 1896. He earmarked the contribution for "the protection of women from cancer." Neely accepted the donation and forwarded it to Dr. Joseph Colt Bloodgood, with instructions that the doctor use the money as Sims had requested.[5]

Bloodgood had trained at the University of Pennsylvania and then joined Johns Hopkins University as a specialist in surgery and cancer. A student of William Halsted's and a founding member of the ASCC, he studied cancer in women and believed that early detection, followed by surgery, could cure cancer. He published extensively on cancer and regularly addressed national audiences on the subject.[6] Neely described Bloodgood as "one of the greatest, if not the greatest cancer surgeon in the world, and one of the most princely men that I have ever had the good fortune to know." Since the 1920s, Bloodgood had consistently provided Neely with the medical and scientific expertise the senator needed to create cancer legislation. Neely trusted Bloodgood and felt confident that Bloodgood would put the Sims donation to good use.[7]

In recognition of the donor, Bloodgood set up a fund appropriately named the Amanda Sims Memorial Fund. He designated the money to support cervical cancer education programs. Specifically, Bloodgood believed that teaching mothers who had recently borne children about the risk of cervical cancer would allow for earlier treatment of the disease and improve treatment outcomes. Convinced that untreated cervical tears contributed to cervical cancer, he wanted to redefine postnatal care so that it included cancer prevention.[8]

Although Bloodgood had earned a reputation within the medical community, he lacked familiarity with women's clubs. In order to advance his theories of preventive examination, he needed to hire a liaison who could promote his medical message to a broad constituency of women. Soon after establishing the ASMF, Bloodgood hired

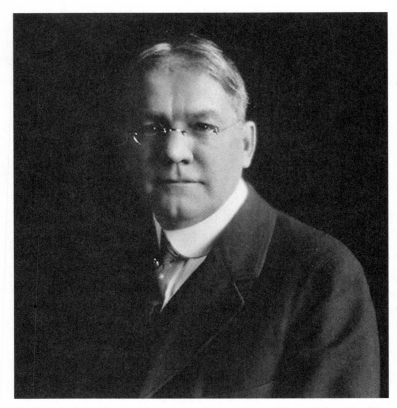

Dr. Joseph Colt Bloodgood (1867–1935), cancer specialist at Johns Hopkins University and founder of the Amanda Sims Memorial Fund and its cervical cancer awareness initiative. (Courtesy of Alan Mason Chesney Medical Archives, Johns Hopkins Medical Institutions, Baltimore, Md.)

Florence Becker, a trained nurse and public health advocate, as his "secretary." A secretary in title only, she designed an educational program that would extend beyond the medical profession and mobilize women's clubs throughout the United States. A privileged woman with years of experience in women's reform work, Becker employed her extensive knowledge of female social networks to attract the cooperation of the General Federation of Women's Clubs (GFWC) and the American Association of University Women (AAUW).

Born in 1878, Florence Serpell Deakins Becker spent much of her adult life committed to health reform. She started school for medical training, but her education was cut short when she decided to work during the Spanish-American War. She nursed typhoid patients during the war, and in 1900 she earned a patent for a particular hospital bed that she designed. She married geologist George F. Becker in 1902, a marriage that lasted until his death in 1919. She continued her medical work throughout this period, volunteering for the Red Cross during World War I. In the 1920s she engaged in tuberculosis control in India and married J. C. Forrester. With the demise of this marriage and the legal battles that accompanied it, Becker left Bombay and returned to the United States in March 1930.[9]

Notes exchanged with friends during this transition indicated that she experienced some difficulty returning to the United States. She felt nostalgic for her public health work and life in India. As she wrote to a friend, "I am giving it [cancer work] as serious consideration as I gave to tuberculosis," but she added that she missed her previous career: "I must admit my heart is on the old work and I long to go back to India and carry on."[10]

After decades of work related to health and health services, Becker now found herself confronting the cancer problem in the United States. In short time, she recognized the potential of an early detection campaign. Her subsequent enthusiasm and dedication to cancer prevention transformed her outlook about her new career and relocation to the United States. Throughout the 1930s Becker recruited women's clubs to support the effort, delivered radio speeches on the subject, edited Bloodgood's public speeches for women's groups, and gained sponsors for cancer awareness material.[11]

Becker brought valuable social connections and public health experience to this job. She organized the ASMF initiative, tapping into numerous networks that could promote cancer awareness. Although she was given multiple titles, including assistant, secretary, and directress, within a year Bloodgood had asked Florence Becker to take charge of the fund, now formally named the "Mrs. Amanda Sims Memorial Fund for the Protection of Mothers from Cancer by Cor-

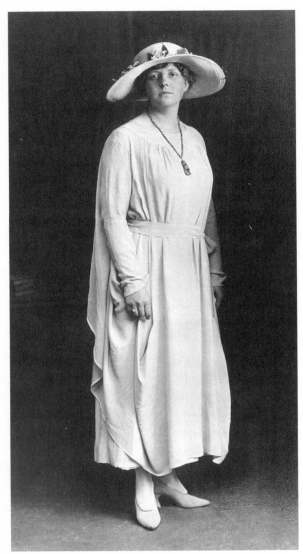

Florence Serpell Deakins Becker (1878–1969). As the director of the Amanda Sims Memorial Fund, Becker networked with dozens of women's clubs to promote cervical cancer awareness. (Library of Congress, Prints and Photographs Division)

rect Information and Periodic Pelvic Examinations." As childbirth became increasingly medicalized in the twentieth century, theories about cervical tears and their connection to cancer gained currency in female audiences, who increasingly deferred to medical expertise in matters of birthing. With this logic and approach, the ASMF initiatives explicitly focused on new mothers.[12]

A little over a year after Becker joined Bloodgood's office, she wrote to a friend, "Every minute of my time has been devoted to the campaign which I have undertaken. The days have been extended until 12 o'clock midnight, and yet I do not get through with the message . . . for the protection of women from cancer by correct information. . . . I have made rather good contacts and we are pushing ahead."[13] Becker's emphasis on sharing this message, making contacts, and "pushing ahead" echoed physicians who endorsed early detection as the key to cancer control. Persuaded by doctor-approved messages of early detection, Becker believed that female networks offered a way to transform a large number of women's lives in a short amount of time by offering vital information about their health and bodies.

From a medical perspective, Bloodgood endorsed female education as a way to reduce reproductive cancer mortality. He expressed concern that the cancer awareness programs initiated in the preceding decades had favored cancers of the breast and skin and thereby had marginalized the risk that reproductive cancers posed to female communities. As he explained it: "While advice in regard to a lump in the breast, or a sore spot in the mouth, or a mole, is likely to be followed, that as regards the unusual discharge goes unheeded. Indeed, often it fails to find its way into print. When information is sent to the press, with few exceptions everything is published except statements in regard to the unusual vaginal discharge. One of the great press organizations has written me frankly that it prefers not to publish the words uterus, cervix, discharge, bloody, or menses."[14] Recognizing the challenges posed by the desire for polite conversation and the need for descriptive language about cancer indications, Bloodgood turned to Becker, an expert in female education, who could consider alternative ways to teach women this medical message.

Like many health professionals, Becker was persuaded by Blood-good's medical opinion, and, like many women involved in the ASCC, she endorsed the idea that early cancer detection offered the best means to a cure.[15] When she turned to women's organizations as a network that could share this information within a broad female community, she took advantage of a history of women's reform work defined by efforts to improve women's lives and society. Becker did not challenge conventional medical wisdom but instead further legitimized it by gaining female support for it. Her education program taught women that regular pelvic examinations in combination with postnatal care offered protection from cervical cancer.[16] Becker confronted a culture that was generally unfamiliar with routine medical exams, and specifically wary of vaginal exams. In 1930 few family physicians or clinics contacted patients regularly, and fewer still considered routine pelvic examinations important for cancer prevention.[17] Although both physicians and patients needed education about contemporary cancer prevention, this campaign initially focused on female patients, specifically mothers. As Bloodgood stated, "the spreading of this important knowledge to the masses depends absolutely upon the women. Women can be frank with one another more so than the average young mother is with a physician."[18]

Becker thus turned to all-female spaces as sites for cancer education. Rather than relying on newsprint and magazine articles, she utilized networks of women. As she explained, "As this is an educational movement by women, with women, and for women, its efficiency and rapidity of progress will depend upon increasing the number of women who understand it and we are willing to help in bringing this message to their own community, their own doctors, and their friends."[19] Employing expressions such as "by women, for women, and with women," Becker fostered a sense of female empowerment in cancer control. Contributing to a professional project that prioritized clinical knowledge, the educational program likewise encouraged women to participate in the medical transformation taking place.

Becker and Bloodgood worked as a team, and their strategies of education and research tended to complement one another. For instance, Becker embraced Bloodgood's medical theories and language of prevention. She encouraged women's organizations to participate in the movement by stressing the value of routine pelvic examinations to all their members. She envisioned ways to broaden her female audience, and her ultimate goals reflected a desire to reach all members of the lay female community and convey her knowledge about the threat of cervical cancer. While Becker focused on liaisons with female audiences and public outreach, Bloodgood devoted most of his energy to medical research in the laboratory, clinic, and hospital. Becker never challenged Bloodgood's expertise; instead, as he advanced his studies of cervical cancers, his convictions gained additional authority.[20]

Although Becker and Bloodgood created a solid partnership that advanced this program of early detection, each espoused a specific goal. Becker focused on women and cervical cancer, measuring the success of the program in the number of women's lives saved. The rhetoric she employed in ASMF publications suggests a burgeoning feminist consciousness about women's health. Bloodgood shared the particular interest in cancers specific to women but failed to appreciate the gendered nature of this problem. For him, cervical cancer was specific to women, and he viewed women as a population group. Further, according to him, women offered a key to the promotion of family health generally. As he explained, "There is much more to this movement for the protection of mothers by correct information and periodic pelvic examinations. The mother's instinct for the protection of her children and the family is greater than the father's."[21] His assumptions concerning gender were not uncommon for this period. He imagined women in the home, as guardians of the nation's health, and as volunteers willing to educate others. His reliance on women to promote health awareness exposed some of the social and cultural trends that allowed women to participate in cancer awareness in the early decades of the twentieth century.

To launch the campaign, Becker invited various women's groups to the home of Mrs. Delos Blodgett in Washington, D.C., on a Thursday afternoon in January 1931.[22] At this informal meeting several women and at least one male doctor gathered to discuss cancer prevention. Participants contributed to the resulting document, an eleven-page statement entitled *The Protection of Women from Cancer: An Educational Program by Women, for Women, with Women.* This unsigned, privately circulated statement consisted of a discussion of contemporary medical and popular understandings of cancer, an outline of treatment options, and a brief review of the cancer education campaign in the United States. The author, or authors, emphasized that current educational efforts did not tackle cervical cancer, a disease many believed could be prevented by early detection.[23] Varying little from traditional cancer awareness literature, the medical information offered in this pamphlet insisted on the value of early detection.[24]

Yet the document also emphasized that women should organize to inform each other about cervical cancer, to teach others about the benefits of regular pelvic examinations, and to spread the message of cervical cancer prevention. As the conclusion stated, "Here is a great opportunity for women to demonstrate that they can protect themselves and ultimately lead in the health and preventive-health movement as well as aiding in medical research."[25] The document stressed the importance of collaboration among individual women, local women's groups, community groups, and larger entities, and it applauded women's ability to popularize health messages. Maintaining a focus on women, the document's authors spoke to female audiences and hoped to convince them to join the cervical cancer awareness campaign. The program outlined contemporary medical understandings of cancer and encouraged women to demand pelvic examinations as preventive treatment. The document simultaneously served women who needed this information and doctors who wanted their theories promulgated to a broader audience. When women increasingly followed this message (and it appears that many women in this community did), they consulted physicians and deferred to their expertise in matters of cancer care. As women advanced cancer education, then, they inadvertently weakened traditional bonds of knowledge that women shared and advanced professional advice as superior knowledge.

Realizing that women's clubs provided an ideal way to reach white middle-class females, Becker championed Bloodgood's theories in letters to influential women in Washington, D.C., leading national women's organizations, and women's clubs. Becker's knowledge of white women's organizations and her familiarity with club work enhanced her ability to involve these groups in cervical cancer awareness. She recruited women from the American Association of University Women, American Red Cross, ASCC, GFWC, League of Women Voters, Women's City Clubs, and the Young Women's Christian Association (YWCA) to join this cancer crusade. The Bureau of Public Health responded to her pleas by carrying on cancer education work in local units.[26]

A case study of the AAUW illustrates the importance of collaborative work among women's organizations in this period. As these discussions between Becker, Bloodgood, and the AAUW reveal, as early as the 1930s powerful women began identifying women's health as a political concern. The discourse employed by the ASMF, which bestowed women with information, attracted support from a broad network of women.

The American Association of University Women

On February 5, 1931, Becker started her correspondence with Dr. Katherine McHale, the AAUW's executive and educational secretary. Becker described cervical cancer education as "an entirely new kind of educational movement. We desire no publicity whatever and we believe that only the individual efforts on the part of women themselves are required, and not money, to prevent the increase of the death rate from cancer."[27] McHale read of Becker's working relationship with Bloodgood and their efforts to organize women, teach female communities about cervical cancer, and inform women about the need for annual pelvic examinations. Within one week of receiving Florence Becker's letter of introduction, McHale responded enthusiastically. McHale's response suggested a willingness to cooperate with Becker and Bloodgood, as well as her desire to support the medical profession. She agreed to publish a medical article by Bloodgood in the AAUW journal, admitting that this journal, which reached an educated female audience, rarely included medical opinions.[28] Recognizing the importance of spreading this message to women, McHale emphasized that the AAUW's membership could dispense information about this new initiative nationwide.[29] She stressed that the AAUW publication reached "thirty-six thousand college women organized into six hundred branches throughout the United States and its territories, and that they represent in their respective communities potential readers with contacts in almost every women's group in the communities."[30]

In an effort to reconcile the needs of her organization with Bloodgood's medical specialty, McHale suggested that Bloodgood explicitly address three issues in his article for the AAUW. Revealing her hands-on approach to health education, familiarity with her audience, and desire to see the effort succeed, McHale assumed an authoritative role as educator when she advised Bloodgood about the most effective way to address this audience.

First, McHale recommended that Bloodgood "approach the subject . . . as a problem in education" in order to make the topic relevant to the AAUW audience. McHale endorsed education as a way to change perceptions of cancer. "Education of the right sort," she explained, "might modify women's psychological attitude toward [cervical cancer and pelvic examinations]."[31] In addition, she approved the information campaign as a way to correct misperceptions or negative images of the disease. Second, McHale believed that the "application of intelligence and understanding" would help instill the habit of regular, preventive pelvic examinations. This comment may allude to Becker's goal of informing women of the medical necessity of examination. McHale rejected health campaigns that dictated behavior protocol without informing the patients about the examination process.[32] Finally, she pondered the idea of "getting women to submit themselves to a complete examination for health reasons." Her choice of the verb "submit" indicated her recognition of the discomfort and vulnerability some women may have experienced during a vaginal exam. McHale wanted to convince women of the dire need for these exams and thoughtfully evaluated the best way to do so. McHale's immediate devotion to this agenda secured the mutually beneficial relationship between the AAUW and the ASMF.[33]

A month later, in March 1931, the AAUW agreed to send each of its members a survey about cervical cancer. These questionnaires asked about the women's knowledge of pelvic examinations. A second section, to be completed by the participants' doctors, asked the physicians how regularly they performed such examinations. The AAUW encouraged its members to answer the questions, collect responses from their doctors, and return both completed surveys to Bloodgood's office. By the next year, the *Journal of the American Association of University Women* reported that 30,000 women had completed the survey.[34] Becker was proud of the AAUW's involvement:

> The American Association of University Women was the first organization to undertake the obligation of teaching their entire membership [about cervical cancer] and of securing the opinion of the family physicians. The work done by this organization has extended into every state in these United States. Many women have answered the circular letter. Over 300 physicians have personally replied to us in answer to the University Women's inquiry, expressing their belief that only through an annual examination can women be protected from developing cancer of the cervix. The printed material distributed by the American Association of University Women has been of educational value to the physicians and laity throughout the United States of America.[35]

Moreover, Bloodgood's article "Cancer Prevention—A Task in Education" appeared in the *Journal of the American Association for University Women* in June 1932. He heeded McHale's advice and tailored the article to educated women. He argued that "developing preventive medicine to its fullest usefulness is chiefly a problem of education" and stressed that cervical cancer detection was part of preventive medicine. Reinforcing the value of female networks, he claimed that individual women could be the best vehicles for this message because "the basic principles and facts of preventive medicine cannot be taught to the people by the press." Bloodgood feared that simple messages conveyed by the media reduced complicated ideas into sound bites and offered instruction without dialogue. Although audiences may have learned from the press, the press could not answer their questions or address individual concerns in the way that women's networks could.[36]

The AAUW continued to publish information about cancer prevention for its members. In its 1932 publication *The Health of Women from Adolescence through Adulthood*, members learned about a wide range of topics including general hygiene, internal medicine, orthopedics, accidents, and preventive measures against disease, including a discussion of cancer. The AAUW publication suggested that education and periodic pelvic examinations offered two ways for women to actively participate in the prevention and treatment of cancer.[37] Moreover, AAUW used its formal network to publicize cancer awareness and prevention information. This approach served as a model for other women's clubs that were interested in increasing women's knowledge of cancer.[38] As one example, a woman eager to join in cancer prevention efforts inquired about ways she might contribute to this national effort. Becker immediately referred her to the AAUW, explaining that the AAUW disseminated health pamphlets to all its members. She encouraged this woman to follow its lead and "influence the Daughters of the American Revolution, The Colonial Dames, The Federation of Women's Clubs, and such groups, recruit more participation from women's clubs, and, not least of all, spread the message of early detection through routine pelvic examinations."[39]

The cooperation evident between the AAUW and the ASMF reflected trends of the 1930s that recognized female cancers as a women's health concern.[40] In an era of growing medical professionalism, the doctrine of early detection placed physicians in the authoritative position for diagnosis. Women learned information about the disease and shared it with other women, then consulted doctors for examinations. Bloodgood praised the work of the AAUW: "The facts in regard to cancer prevention have been presented to the American Association of University Women before, and no group of either men or women have responded more effectively than university women."[41] As a result of this collaboration, the ASMF proved that tapping into established networks of women could broaden the audience and impact of cancer awareness efforts.

In its early years, the ASMF followed a specific agenda that tended to reach mothers who lived in the Northeast. It focused exclusively on cervical cancer awareness, and its audience was generally privileged women, with higher educations, as exemplified by its relationship with the AAUW. Although primarily limited to middle-class and white women, this early cervical cancer education campaign provided women with medical information, explicitly reminding audiences that women could teach one another about cancer and participate in medical programs. They encouraged women to engage in dialogue with medical experts by simple practices such as collecting the survey cards and by more direct actions that encouraged women to insist on preventive exams. The ASMF trusted the impact of women's organizations and networks to convey this information to audiences far and wide. Dr. Bloodgood, and undoubtedly other physicians, benefited from women's involvement in early cancer awareness campaigns. The educational program informed women, but it also served physicians by advancing their medical opinions and advice. Moreover, it reinforced notions of individual responsibility and cancer care, implicitly placing a burden on mothers to seek additional medical consultation after childbirth.

Influencing Health Policy

Throughout the early 1930s the ASMF continued to broaden its audience by recruiting additional women's organizations to promote cervical cancer awareness. The American Red Cross distributed cancer literature in rural areas and promised that eight hundred public health nurses would distribute additional cervical cancer detection information. The League of Women Voters endorsed regular cervical examinations; Women's City Clubs sponsored speeches on the subject; and the YWCA revised its health manual to include recommendations for vaginal exams. Furthermore, the YWCA equipped various centers so that the vaginal examinations could be conducted there. Finally, the GFWC, with membership that exceeded 300,000 women, supported these educational efforts.

Records from the early years of the ASMF indicate that Becker organized a letter-writing campaign to encourage women to become politically active. She urged McHale to write her congressional representative to insist that he support preventative health measures. As Becker explained, "Congress could pass a resolution authorizing the National Institute of Health to take up the problem of providing the people with correct information in regard to all matters of preventive medicine and health."[42] Placing cancer within the larger context of preventive health care would ensure more funding for awareness programs. She further encouraged McHale and others to work within their states to convince governors to mandate changes in local health departments, part of her explicit attempt to politicize her base of supporters.

Becker also worked on promoting cervical cancer education beyond the United States.[43] She asked friends as far away as London and Calcutta to spread the message. Becker had met most of these friends during her career in tuberculosis work, and many were already involved in health crusades and women's groups. In one letter to a friend in London, Becker wrote, "It [cervical cancer educational effort] is done entirely by personal contact, seeing and talking my head off and not asking for money. Consequently most of the women have listened to me. I believe you could do the same thing in England among your large group of hearers."[44] In a letter to Colonel Hugh William Acton, a professor at the School of Tropical Medicine in Calcutta, Becker wrote, "I am now organizing an educational campaign the telling [to] every woman who has borne a child that it is absolutely vital she go to a physician of reputable standing at least once a year and have a thorough pelvic examination. . . . I enclose you a pamphlet which you can read, and if you consider it advisable to distribute I will send you more." Informed by Bloodgood's conviction that cervical tears could cause cancer, Becker's awareness program was still directed at a narrow audience of mothers, even as its geographical scope was extended.[45]

As the ASMF expanded its reach, it also developed a working relationship with the ASCC, the largest cancer society in the United States. Both groups shared common concerns, and by 1932, the ASCC generously offered to send its printed material on female cancer to the 587 branches of the AAUW.

The emerging alliance reflected common goals among these organizations, as well as the significant inroads made by the ASMF. The ASCC wanted access to the female audiences identified by the ASMF. As an ASCC staff member explained to the AAUW, "This society will be most happy to cooperate with your organization and with Dr. Bloodgood in any way we can. We take it that you will let us know at a later date how we may best do this—either by sending you a supply of our literature, or by sending us the names and addresses of the various branches which wish to have kit packages of our literature."[46] The ASCC, which was already informed by Bloodgood's ideas, endorsed the ASMF message that regular pelvic examinations offered the best way to detect cervical cancer in its early stages and incorporated this message into its publications and statements. Evidently, there was little to no hostility between the ASCC and the ASMF, and each maintained its distinct mission in the early 1930s. In fact, years later, AAUW president Katherine McHale filled leadership roles for the ASCC, serving on the National Advisory Council of the Women's Field Army between 1936 and 1938.

It is impossible to isolate the impact of the ASMF in an era when various cancer education programs succeeded, but clearly this campaign offered a model for promoting cancer awareness exclusively through women's groups. The ASMF message—that regular pelvic examinations offered the best protection for women—was endorsed by the ASCC. The partnership of Becker and Bloodgood lasted from 1930 until Bloodgood's death in 1935. By then, the fund had been depleted, and many of the initiatives introduced by the ASMF had been fully adopted by the ASCC. The lasting legacy of the Amanda Sims Memorial Fund included increased attention to early indications of cervical cancer, a push to inform women and doctors about medical procedures that enabled early detection, and a reliance on women's clubs to spread information about cancers specific to women. Many of these goals were represented in an alternative organization that likewise emerged in an effort to expand female awareness about cancer, the Women's Field Army.

The General Federation of Women's Clubs

Throughout the 1930s the General Federation of Women's Clubs actively promoted public health programs in the United States. It encouraged its members to learn about state health departments and state medical departments, to protect health appropriations, to support legislation for public health, and to organize community health studies.[47] As Marjorie Illig, chair of the GFWC Division of Public Health, announced to her members in the early 1930s, "THE NATION'S WOMANHOOD MUST DEFEND THE NATION'S HEALTH." The GFWC urged its members to protest the health budget cuts evident in many communities in the early 1930s and to support health programs.[48]

In April 1933, when the GFWC Public Health and Child Welfare Advisory Committee held its second meeting at national headquarters in Washington, D.C., ASCC president Clarence Cook Little approached the organization about considering the creation of a cooperative cancer program.[49] Already committed to the principles of health education, the advisory committee recommended that the GFWC join this effort in order that "the importance of education in the early diagnosis and treatment of cancer be brought to the attention of women of the county." The committee assigned this task to the Public Health Division.[50]

The Public Health Division launched a cancer education program, and by November 1933, the General Federation Advisory Board adopted this program as one of two new initiatives for the year. (The second was a community health study.) Created in cooperation with the ASCC, the education program promoted the message, "Cancer Thrives on Ignorance, Fight It with Knowledge." The Public Health Division printed the cancer education program, forwarded it to all the state federation chairs, and requested that they forward the program directives to clubs. The program emphasized the risk that cancer posed, particularly to women, and insisted that cancer control could be accomplished with simple measures of early detection.[51]

The GFWC employed many of themes that it had used in health promotion throughout the decade, which linked women's health to the strength of the nation. As it explained in the introductory materials, which defined cancer as "the outstanding menace" to women, "The preservation of the health of women in the prime of life is the greatest single guarantee of national stability and successful insurance for home life." The program urged every clubwoman to inform herself about cancer, share this information with friends and family, and support the establishment of cancer facilities that worked toward better education, diagnosis, and treatment. The GFWC started a Cancer Control Fund to offer economic support for these endeavors and asked each member to donate a dime to this fund.[52]

The GFWC recognized the courtesy and cooperation of the ASCC in its year-end notes. In reciprocation, the ASCC invited the chair of the Public Health Division, Marjorie Illig, to attend the annual ASCC meeting in New York City in March 1934, paying all her expenses. Impressed with the meeting, Illig reported, "The sessions were most interesting and inspiring, and conducive to stimulating more enthusiastic and active support in cancer education."[53]

The cancer education program continued in 1934–35. As the Public Health Division recounted, "With increased suffering and death from cancer—particularly among women—it seemed appropriate that clubwomen should shoulder the responsibility of promoting a nation-wide campaign against the disease." The GFWC reported success in creating cancer education programs in nearly every state and in raising over $1,000 for the Cancer Control Fund, concluding, "Interest and enthusiasm in the campaign have gained momentum constantly."[54] The GFWC's sustained interest in cancer control pleased ASCC president Clarence Cook Little. In 1936 he invited the club-women to cooperate more closely with the ASCC by creating a women's division within the ASCC. The WFA welcomed members of the GFWC, offered them leadership positions, and promised that they would play key roles in the fight against cancer. Clubwomen thus learned about "this outstanding menace to the human race—and in particular to women in the prime of life." Finally, they were asked to "carry a message of hope to men and women in every section of this country."[55]

Little's commitment to the WFA reflected several trends that had been evident in cancer reform since the early decades of the twentieth century. First, the ASCC valued women as liaisons who would deliver a message created by the medical profession to lay audiences. As such, the ASCC recognized women's power within communities, especially among networks of women, and believed that women were the perfect agents to usher in a transformation in American culture. Likewise, women concerned about cancer found an outlet in the WFA. Second, women assumed positions of leadership in cancer education, even when dealing with the male-dominated fields of medicine and cancer research. In the WFA women occupied positions that ranged from national field commander to state commander to field officers. Although these women did not challenge the conventional wisdom of medical professionals, they created cancer awareness programs that defined the disease for popular American audiences. Placing enormous emphasis on female and individual responsibility, WFA women taught audiences that they could confront this dreaded disease and play a critical role in health care. Finally, women had a history of voluntarism that would be essential to any reform efforts of the ASCC, which was continually operating on a limited budget.

The GFWC was a good fit for the newly conceived Women's Field Army. Since the turn of the century, the GFWC had worked on sanitation and health issues. Soon thereafter, it had engaged in disease-specific work focused on tuberculosis control. When C. C. Little of the ASCC approached the organization in 1933, he hoped that women would contribute to the society's effort to inform the public about the disease and encourage prompt response to any cancer suspicions. As a GFWC historian recounted, the ASCC explained that "if women learned the truth about means for its [cancer's] control and spoke out on the subject, then lives would be saved by early detection of the disease."[56] Reinforcing the idea that cancer could be cured, the ASCC, the WFA, and the GFWC all emphasized individual responsibility in early cancer detection. Popular cancer rhetoric insisted that individual patients, most specifically women, needed to learn about early cancer detection, to teach others about it, and comply with medical guidelines. As reported in the *New York Times*, "Because women are not only guardians of the family's health but are themselves, more often than men the prey to cancer, they have been drafted under the banner of the American Society for the Control of Cancer to do the work."[57]

Little, who had been eager to create a cooperative cancer program that formally recruited women to the ASCC, cemented the relationship with the GFWC by hiring Marjorie Illig, chair of the GFWC Public Health Division, to be the national commander of the WFA, an appointment formalized by 1937. Illig, a leader of and expert in women's clubs, would ensure the quick and effective recruitment of women to cancer awareness. Moreover, the ASCC budgeted $5,000 for Illig's salary. Adding Illig to the ASCC payroll indicated a departure in cancer awareness, which had depended on female voluntary labor for decades.[58] Grace Morrison Poole, GFWC president, agreed to serve as the chief adviser of the WFA.[59] In addition, members of the GFWC served as state commanders throughout the nation.

By the late 1930s, the WFA adopted the motto that women would "fight cancer with knowledge" and acted as an independent agency within the ASCC. Women assumed positions and titles in this organization whose structure reflected that of the military. The WFA designed programs for exclusively female audiences that discussed breast and reproductive cancers, and it also offered general programs on cancer that affected men, women, and children.

The GFWC played a vital role in sustaining the WFA. An umbrella organization that included hundreds of national women's clubs, the GFWC was one of the most influential organizations to result from the reform era. The GFWC facilitated the WFA's goals by offering financial assistance to patients in need, establishing diagnostic centers, and directing additional financial support to cancer research. When the ASCC secured the support of the GFWC, it gained important economic and political clout. Moreover, the support of eminent leaders Illig and Poole, who agreed with the premise that cancer education would bring about a cancer cure, ensured national cooperation in this effort.[60]

The Women's Field Army

In 1937, after several years of planning, the WFA launched a nationwide campaign to promote cancer education and expand its membership. With members working in thirty states, it set up booths in railway stations and more, fostering cancer-consciousness among the public and appealing to individuals to do their part against cancer.[61] In a very short time, the WFA made lasting impressions on public perceptions of cancer.

The Women's Field Army worked to "more effectively and unitedly fight Cancer." ASCC president Clarence Cook Little's explanation about why the society created a women's army reflected the gendered norms of this era. Women would be the leaders of cancer education, he argued, "because the types of cancer that strike women hardest—cancer of the uterus and breast—may be cured in seventy per cent of the cases if taken in time. Because women are the natural guardians of the family's health. Because women have played a splendid role in combating tuberculosis and in charity and public health drives."[62] Little employed the pervasive assumption that women, who were constantly positioned vis-à-vis a family, needed to learn basic tools for maintaining health among all family members. He recognized women's historic contributions to public health campaigns by noting women's experience with tuberculosis control. The ASCC would similarly rely on women to further its goals of cancer control.

Remarkably, this all-female branch of the ASCC assumed an organizational style that imitated the military, a bastion of masculinity. The military references served at least three purposes. First, they alluded to the active fight against cancer and the need for aggressive responses to it.[63] Second, they allowed women to assume ranks and leadership roles in a formal organization. Unlike the ASCC, which tended to limit women's access to leadership, the WFA encouraged women to lead this educational campaign. Finally, the borrowed imagery, though almost exclusively male, was imbued with power and authority. Endorsed by the medical profession and the ASCC, the armylike structure never became a mockery of inverted gender roles. Instead, it allowed women limited authority and elicited public recognition of this authority through visual markers of power, including military-style uniforms, titles, and honors.

The WFA, also referred to as the "educational arm of the ASCC," displayed its members' ranking and listed chains of command. Members wore brown uniforms with insignia that designated the specific rank. Marjorie Illig assumed the role of national commander, the highest position in the WFA. Other national leadership positions included honorary appointments and membership in the executive committee. The WFA organized branches in each state, under the leadership of a state commander. Representatives of the state medical societies, state health departments, the ASCC, and select laypersons made up the state advisory and executive committees, which acted as umbrella organizations for all state programs. Finally, the WFA was divided into local branches that included local advisory and executive committees, local captains, and nonranking members or the "soldiers of the field." While membership fluctuated, in any given year several hundred thousand women belonged to the WFA.[64]

The highly defined and organized structure of the WFA provided unambiguous positions for women working within the organization.

Members were tasked with various goals that ranged from the promotion of cancer education to the recruitment of new members. The military-like structure may have lent an authenticity to this division of labor as well. As Barron Lerner has described, cancer education programs frequently adopted metaphors of war. By adopting the formality of military structure, the WFA placed itself in the forefront of those committed to fighting cancer.[65]

The WFA had ambitious goals, ultimately hoping to enlist every American woman in its cancer crusade. Unlike the Sims program, which focused solely on cervical cancer, the Women's Field Army spread information about all cancers and informed both men and women about the risk of the disease. Women could join the WFA, or as the promotional literature read, "enlist in the Army," for a one-time fee of one dollar. Membership fees supplemented the WFA budget, which allocated 70 percent of its funds to the state chapters, 20 percent to its headquarters in New York City, and 10 percent to a contingency fund.[66] Within one year of its formation, the WFA had recruited over 100,000 members; and while it is impossible to know its peak enrollment, it exceeded 300,000 members. Some periodicals even suggested that membership exceeded 700,000 before it was absorbed into the American Cancer Society in 1945.[67]

The WFA maintained a close relationship with medical professionals, explicitly seeking their approval for programming and often inviting physicians to serve on its committees. (Men could also contribute financially to the WFA but could not enlist in the field army.) The articulated goals of the WFA included the expansion of educational initiatives; the creation of more diagnostic and treatment centers; provisions for greater financial assistance for all in need; and ultimately, an increase in funding for research initiatives. The early detection program followed guidelines similar in scope to the ASMF. It stressed early detection and subsequent treatment. Also like the ASMF, the WFA reinforced the emerging medical paradigms that suggested that early treatment would increase the rate of cures, popularizing medical ideas for a lay and female audience.

Similar to the AAUW and its immediate support of cervical cancer awareness through the ASMF, the GFWC enthusiastically endorsed the ASCC's idea of promoting cancer education and volunteerism among its female membership. Illig placed cancer awareness within the GFWC's public health campaign, and even before the formal creation of the WFA, the GFWC listed cancer awareness as one of its three most important priorities. Recognizing cancer as a leading concern in the early 1930s, the federation generated broad support for ASCC programs.[68] According to the GFWC, cancer ranked as one of the two greatest diseases (along with syphilis) of the early twentieth century. As Illig explained, "Progress in mastering these two great disease problems *will* be slow until there is general understanding on the part of the public of the principles involved. Control measures are known and have been put to test in scientific circles which when applied in society at large will lead to very great advance toward the final elimination of these destroyers of human life and happiness."[69]

The WFA's basic messages could be summarized in three points. First, the WFA taught that cancer could be cured. Second, it stressed that early detection worked and facilitated successful treatment. Third, it emphasized the necessity of periodic medical examinations, even when a person felt well. All three points reflected the dominant medical opinion. The WFA distinguished between the role of the lay and medical volunteer, encouraging the former to organize speeches, advertisements, and recruitment and the latter to answer queries about the scientific aspects of cancer.

The GFWC, and other all-female networks, helped the WFA fulfill many of its goals, especially the education of large female audiences. However, it also served larger trends in the professionalization of medicine. Although women learned about their bodies and cancer symptoms, cancer awareness material also directed women to defer to medical opinions, to participate in regular medical exams, and, through their actions, to legitimate the merits of contemporary medicine. Although science could not cure cancer, educational literature insisted that the public could combat the disease. For instance, GFWC publications listed cancer awareness as a duty for every clubwoman; she should learn cancer symptoms, examine herself, and visit a physician regularly.[70]

Like the ASCC, the WFA headquarters were located in New York City, and much of the activity of the WFA occurred in the Northeast. Not surprisingly, the New York City Cancer Committee (NYCCC) played a leading role in creating the WFA. Founded in 1926, the NYCCC was a self-supporting local branch of the ASCC that focused on distributing messages of early detection and prompt treatment. By 1936, it had organized a national recruitment week every spring to recruit new members to its organization. The NYCCC sponsored publications, and especially the production of pamphlets, that could be distributed to various gatherings of women.[71]

One of the most telling pamphlets of the era, *There Shall Be Light!*, was published in 1936 and offered readers contemporary facts about cancer while celebrating the accomplishments of the ASCC. The cover of the pamphlet featured a sword, upright, in the front and center. Dozens of women lined up behind the sword, symbolizing the army of volunteers who were fighting cancer. Relying on the metaphor of war, this image captured the vigilance of many female cancer activists. The sword represented the tool that might battle the enemy, and the women literally represented the soldiers who would employ the sword. The combination of masculine and feminine imagery captured the involvement of women, even in traditionally defined masculine spaces and organizations. Sponsored by two generous and anonymous donors, this pamphlet explicitly described the goals of the WFA as educational.

The pamphlet, distributed widely during recruitment week, mirrored most ASCC publications in its inclusion of information about the disease, emphasis on early diagnosis, and suggestion for immediate surgical treatment. "The purpose of this campaign is to spread as far as possible among women, who are the chief sufferers, the message that Cancer Can Be Cured If Promptly Treated," the pamphlet announced. However, in its deliberate effort to attract women, the pamphlet also told the history of women's contributions to female cancer awareness, stressing their roles in medical research, philanthropy, and volunteerism.[72]

To this special end, *There Shall Be Light* featured biographical sketches of women in medical research, including Drs. Marie Curie, Maud Slye, Elise L'Esperance, and Elizabeth Hurdon. Madame Curie discovered radium, a cancer therapy widely used by the 1930s. She had received support for her work with radium from the ASCC, and the pamphlet featured a picture of Curie with a leading ASCC advocate, Elise Mead. Maud Slye's research on cancer and heredity was also celebrated. Dr. Elizabeth Hurdon opened the first hospital for the treatment of cancer in women in London, and several years later, in 1932, Dr. Elise L'Esperance opened a similar clinic, named the Kate Depew Strang Clinic, for women in New York City. L'Esperance and her sister, May Strang, founded this hospital in memory of their mother.[73]

Women's participation in cancer philanthropy was also commemorated in this booklet. The publication identified the leading female donors in cancer research, including Mrs. John Jacob Astor, Mrs. George W. Cullum, and Mrs. Collis P. Huntington. Mrs. Astor and Mrs. Cullum had donated money for the creation of the first cancer hospital in the United States, Memorial Hospital in New York City, founded in 1884. Mrs. Huntington established a cancer research fund and built the Huntington Memorial Hospital in Boston for cancer research.[74]

Finally, *There Shall Be Light* highlighted the achievements of women involved in the ASCC, including Elise Mead and Gertrude Clark. Mead's participation in the ASCC dated back to its creation, and she had continually served the ASCC in a variety of capacities. She sat on the Ways and Means Committee, served as the chair of finance for the NYCCC, and acted as chair of the Women's Committee of the NYCCC. Clark had long served the New York Skin and Cancer Hospital and began working for the NYCCC in 1928.[75]

While highlighting the medical, philanthropic, and voluntary contributions of women, WFA publications and programs promoted an overall knowledge of cancer and often featured details about early

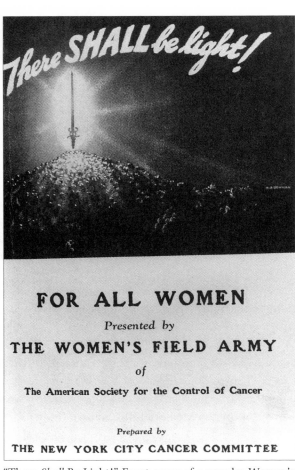

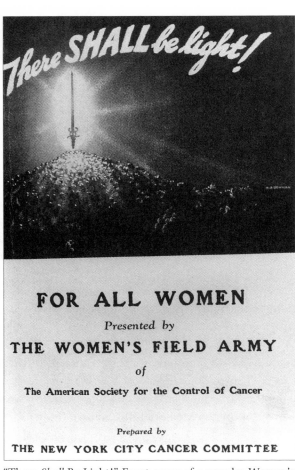

FOR ALL WOMEN

Presented by

THE WOMEN'S FIELD ARMY

of

The American Society for the Control of Cancer

Prepared by

THE NEW YORK CITY CANCER COMMITTEE

"There *Shall* Be Light!" Front cover of a popular Women's Field Army publication, 1936. (Courtesy of the American Cancer Society)

cases of breast and uterine cancer. Likely influenced by the work of the ASMF, the WFA encouraged postpartum examinations and repair of cervical tears, warning that tears left untreated might become cancerous. In addition to toeing the line of the dominant, and largely male, medical profession, the WFA singled out *female* physicians, describing them as beneficial to its agenda: "the woman physician has a special responsibility in these cases [of breast and cervical cancers] because of the greater willingness of many women to submit to examination by one of their own sex." Although some educational components stressed traditional gender roles, particularly evident in references to women in the home, other aspects of the campaign recognized the importance of women's participation in health-care decisions. Recognizing that female physicians could play key roles in this campaign reinforced their gender but also legitimized their place in a profession where women were frequently marginalized.[76] A second WFA pamphlet reiterated this idea when it described the Kate Depew Strang Clinic in New York as a hospital staffed by women who specialized in cancer detection and female physicians who studied the disease.[77] Finally, WFA literature also recognized the nurse and social worker as significant actors in cancer awareness. The WFA believed they had "the advantage of intimate relationship with the patient, even more so than the doctor" and therefore were "more apt to be consulted regarding small lumps in the breast or irregular bleeding."[78]

Venues as diverse as newspapers and popular magazines, billboard advertisements, and bus and subway cards offered the public information about this female branch of the ASCC. Cancer bulletins also directed women to ASCC offices, clinics, and doctors' offices with assurances that a female staff and support network could assist and advise anyone concerned about cancer. A typical advertisement conveyed a limited amount of information but frequently invited the reader to visit a local ASCC office. Because female volunteers staffed most offices, the WFA presented the local ASCC office as a small meeting space for women to privately discuss concerns about their bodies and health. "At any of these offices," one pamphlet claimed, "one can talk confidentially of symptoms and also of personal finances."[79] It seems likely that as early as the mid-1930s, prior to visiting a physician, women discussed cancer among themselves.

By 1937, when Eleanor Roosevelt headed its national advisory board, the WFA had won the endorsement of the National Organization of Public Health Nurses, the Association of Women in Public Health, the National Association of Colored Women, the National Federation of Business and Professional Women, Zonta International, the National Council of Jewish Women, the International Federation of Business and Professional Women, Daughters of the American Revolution, the National Woman's Relief Society, the American Association of University Women, and the Catholic Daughters of America, as well as the continued support of the General Federation of Women's Clubs.[80] Politicians offered accolades to the WFA for its achievements. As Senator Homer Truett Bone (D.-Wash.) proclaimed in 1937, "An organization of which Mrs. Franklin D. Roosevelt is a leader is calling public attention to the fact that cancer is no longer entirely incurable; that radium, x-ray, and the knife can conquer this malignant growth if recognized in time; that there is no reason for the victim of this disease to cover the fact as though it were something to be ashamed of."[81]

Similarly, in the late 1930s Representative Edith Nourse Rogers (R.-Mass.) stated, "Women everywhere in this country are becoming more and more interested in the subject. The field army is consolidating this interest and showing them how to use it constructively in the war that must be fought against the insidious menace. The organized women of America can do much to drive the scourge from the land." Rogers praised the work of the WFA: "This is one of the finest movements ever instituted for the relief of suffering humanity."[82] She recorded her endorsement of the organization, its work, and its concern for women and cancer in the *Congressional Record*. Long committed to recognizing the contributions of women, Rogers legitimized their work further by listing the names of the WFA leaders, acknowledging their expertise and background in public health, and asking Congress to support WFA programs. "It is the first organized campaign against cancer," she argued; "To win, it must have the active cooperation of each one of us. We must stop this alarming increase in cancer deaths."[83]

In 1938 Rogers introduced a resolution that asked Congress to designate April as "cancer control month," as another way to support the WFA's efforts to educate the public about cancer. Rogers supported congressional funding for cancer research, referring to it as "a very meritorious measure." Along with large financial appropriations to cancer research, Rogers stressed, cancer education offered a necessary complement to cancer research. Her proposal reminded Congress of the WFA's and the ASCC's educational mission and the history of women's involvement in this crusade. Moreover, women were particularly susceptible to cancer, as Rogers pointed out: "The estimate of the medical authorities that 300,000 women in this country have cancer is a challenge to each and every one of us." As she articulated, "The Women's Field Army, headed by the able Mrs. Grace Morrison Poole, is doing its part by reaching out into the women's clubs and organizations, obtaining their interest and cooperation in bringing into the open the thousands and thousands of cases which are hidden through fear and terror. It is great work, and unselfish, charitable task. If this Congress can help in it, if by any act of Congress, can lend its hand in assistance, I know it will do so."[84]

The creation of the WFA in the mid-1930s and the autonomy it granted to women within the ASCC speak to the complicated history of women's participation in cancer control efforts throughout the first half of the twentieth century. Despite formal recognition of women's participation in education and reform, as evidenced by Illig's salary and Little's concerted recruitment of women within the GFWC, the WFA was embedded within a patriarchal system of medical expertise. Most notable, the ASCC insisted that each new local branch of the WFA gain the support of local medical societies, which were dominated by male leadership. Although women were encouraged to enroll additional members, men ultimately made decisions about the expansion of the WFA. Moreover, the WFA propagated the ASCC's simple message that concentrated on early detection and prompt response and never challenged conventional medical wisdom.

Did the patriarchy evident within the ASCC, and within medicine more generally, undermine the agency of women within the WFA? My research suggests that women supported conventional medical claims not out of mere deference, but rather so that they might participate in cancer control. Emphasis on early detection offered a sound

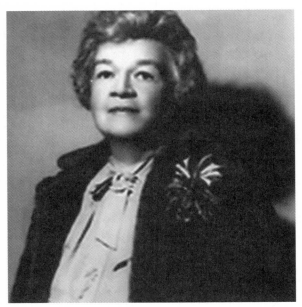

Congresswoman Edith Nourse Rogers (1881–1960). Rogers supported legislation for cancer research and served in honorary positions for the Women's Field Army. (Library of Congress)

medical theory, endorsed by a majority of specialists in the United States, including Drs. Catherine Macfarlane and Elise L'Esperance. It also offered a mechanism for women to respond to this terrifying disease. In the 1930s, not unlike today, laywomen had limited options for combating cancer. Participating in cancer control allowed women to teach one another about disease and female bodies, to respond to personal concerns about cancer, and to contribute to notions of progress against the disease.

The willingness to endorse conventional medical doctrine on cancer reflected a cooperative impulse between voluntary associations and the medical profession. Both the WFA and the ASCC shared the goal of transmitting messages of early detection to female audiences. I have found no evidence to suggest that women differed in their views or that male authorities tried to silence their alternative opinions. Rather, in the early twentieth century, women combined conventional medical advice with their individual experiences with cancer.

False Optimism

Whether orchestrated by the popular press, the ASCC, the ASMF, the WFA, or the federal government, popular cancer education campaigns claimed that the effectiveness of surgery and treatment depended entirely on the stage of diagnosis. Educational material rarely addressed the failures of this theory of early detection, its obvious limitations, or what some critics perceived as its false message of cancer cures.[85] Although intended to replace fear with optimism, the cancer education campaign assured women that early detection would prevent death. Indeed, it often suggested that radical surgery offered a cure and failed to explain the high rate of metastasis and the low rate of long-term survival. Although some critics expressed their views plainly and asked doctors either to demonstrate a cure or to stop laying claim to a cure, others offered subtler criticisms.

In 1937 popular author and novelist Mary Hastings Bradley published a book of fiction entitled *Pattern of Three* that implicitly countered the false optimism of the cancer education campaigns.[86] The plot included the familiar story of a love triangle. Dick, a handsome and powerful lawyer, deserts his supportive wife, Eve, because he has fallen in love with his young and attractive secretary, Kay. In a scenario that reads like a modern soap opera, Dick and Eve divorce, Dick and Kay marry, and then Eve learns she might have breast cancer. As she explains to Dick:

> "I don't want a soul in here to know." She took out a cigarette and held a lighter to it, waving back a match. She said, blowing out a wreath of smoke, "It's annoying—I've got to have something done to me."

He looked at her. "You mean you're ill."

"Not ill. I don't feel a thing. But there's something growing—one of those breast things."

She spoke with such lightness that for a moment he could not realize the seriousness of what she was saying. Her words seemed to be written with the faintest possible legibility on his consciousness. Then, intensely shocked, he made it real.

"You mean you have to be operated upon?"[87]

Capturing central tenets of cancer education in the 1930s, the scene opens with a woman's sense of modesty, or perhaps shame, that she may have breast cancer. The scene also emphasizes the peculiarity of cancer, a deadly disease, whose initial symptoms are not associated with illness.

Eve explains that the lump in her breast might only be a cyst, insists that the surgery (whether a biopsy or mastectomy) is safe, and calms Dick by informing him that the only danger she faces—if the growth proves malignant—is recurrence. When Dick asks Eve why she does not want to tell her friends, Eve explains, "Oh, it's such a horrid operation. One hates—being mutilated." Dick reacts with sympathy: "He thought of her breast being cut into or taken away and compassion was quick in him."[88]

This novel is clearly melodramatic, and the breast cancer story, unlike cancer education films, was not meant to teach a lesson about early detection. Instead, breast cancer offered a literary tool that reflected popular knowledge about cancer and elicited feelings of sympathy from the reader. The information Bradley provides about Eve's breast cancer diagnosis and treatment echoed contemporary understandings of diagnosis and treatment, information commonly printed in women's magazines, WFA literature, and public health bulletins. Unlike the cancer information that overwhelmingly focused on early detection, however, this novel recognized the uncertainty of a cancer diagnosis, even after an early discovery of cancer symptoms. In addition, it acknowledged the disfigurement caused by "mutilating" treatment. Finally, and perhaps most noteworthy, this 1937 narrative reflected a frank discussion of breast cancer and the personal and emotional issues surrounding a potential diagnosis. Women discussed cancer, and many understood its consequences in the 1930s, but few public conversations alluded to mastectomy. In this popular novel by a well-known novelist, Eve speaks frankly about surgery and even conveys a sense of injustice and misogyny when discussing the "mutilating" surgery.[89] Ultimately, the novel traces Eve's death from breast cancer, which Bradley portrays as sad but unsurprising:

> My Dear Dick:
> This is not a letter of good news—at least not for me. You may remember that I had an operation last October. I did not expect any developments so soon—in fact, I was led to believe that there would be none at all. I think I was purposely misled, that I might enjoy these months without any apprehension.
> Now the thing has come back—lower down. The doctor tried to tell me that this new trouble may be something else, independent of the other, something like gall stones, but I know better, I had too much experience with Aunt Margaret not to know what to expect.
> I know this is the end. They want me to go to the hospital. Nothing will happen for several months, I suppose, nothing very definite, I mean, except that I should get weaker and weaker and have to be dosed for the pain. I take only aspirin now. Aunt Margaret went slowly. My case may be quicker. I thought I better write you while I could; there are arrangements I ought to make. I feel so far away. If I am able I shall come home—I want to die at home.[90]

Bradley's character's preparation for death was not a typical scenario in the cancer awareness messages promulgated by the ASMF, the WFA, or the ASCC. In fact, Bradley's open discussion offered a more complex picture of the breast cancer patient than the orchestrated messages of these formal cancer education programs. It explored a woman's sense of mutilation, the risk of metastasis and her fear of this outcome, and the issues of death and dying that accompanied many cancer diagnoses. In an era before informed consent, Eve acknowledges physicians' efforts to deceive her. Eve's experiential knowledge of cancer, gained from her familiarity with Aunt Margaret, suggests the alternative ways that women learned about cancer in the 1930s. In this popular novel genre, the ending proves bittersweet. Before dying, Eve finds solace in her friendship with her husband and his new wife. The husband and wife welcome Eve into their home so that she can indeed "die at home."

A 1940 film, produced by the ASCC in cooperation with U.S. Public Health Service, offers a more typical cancer drama of this era. Like most ASCC productions, this film emphasized the value of early detection and prompt treatment. It also indicated the increased cooperation between the government, the ASCC, and the WFA throughout the late 1930s and early 1940s. This black-and-white, eighteen-minute sound film, *Choose to Live*, tells the story of Mrs. Brown, a white, middle-class housewife who fears she might have cancer. Meant to depict female normalcy in this era, the narrator describes Brown: "Like millions of other women, life revolves around her husband and children, her club, and her friends. Like millions of other mothers, love for her children is equaled only by her responsibility for their welfare."[91]

In its opening scene the film takes the viewer to Washington, D.C., and zooms in on the face of the surgeon general of the U.S. Public Health Service, Thomas Parran. He says, "The American people through their elected representatives of Congress have determined to wage unremitting warfare against cancer." Parran represents an authoritative masculine medical professional committed to combating cancer. Meanwhile, the narrator recites cancer statistics in a somber tone, describing the disease as the second-leading cause of death, no respecter of persons, and the killer of one in every ten individuals.

The film then returns to the narrative by shifting to a domestic scene that surveys Brown's home. Just in case the visual domestic references elude the viewer, the gendered norm of Mrs. Brown as a mother who stays home and cares for the family becomes more explicit. As Brown silently performs her domestic chores, the narrator explains, "She feels perfectly healthy, yet is desperately afraid. She has told no one of her fears, not even her husband. But lurking behind her every act is the ceaseless ebb and flow of her unspoken worry. It can't be. It is. It can't be. It is. To go on with the ordinary day-by-day duties and engagements with this dread always hanging over her. What else is there to do?" The indecisiveness that reverberates in Brown's mind reinforces an emerging motif—female characters who fail to respond immediately to suspicious cancer symptoms are putting their lives at risk. Equating female indecision with immaturity and confusion, the film belittles the main character, whose actions are portrayed as foolish.

Brown eventually attends a local women's club lecture, featuring a noted physician and cancer specialist, where Brown and the viewer learn more about cancer symptoms. The constant messages throughout the film, ranging from Parran's opening advice to the narrator's warnings, echo in the viewer's mind, and the viewer becomes convinced that Brown's life hangs on her attentiveness to her suspicious health problems.

The mounting tension within the film eases as the scene shifts to the physician's lecture, "The Challenge of Cancer." A significant portion of the film is devoted to the depiction of science laboratories, technology, and clinics. Describing cancer as "lawless," the result of "rebellious cells," and the cause of "needless deaths," the film promises that modern science is creating new weapons against the dreaded disease. The physician explores cancer research, cancer treatment, and cancer education. He talks about the continued designation of April as cancer control month, government funding of major cancer research institutions, namely the National Institute of Health and National Cancer Institute, and U.S. Public Health Service efforts to direct more attention to the disease. He emphasizes the potential of science and "new weapons for the war against cancer." He compares physicians, surgeons, and radiologists to soldiers in the war against cancer who will use these new weapons. The physician finally reviews three recommended treatments: surgery, x-ray, and radium.

Now directing his attention to the audience, the doctor urges viewers to have annual cancer exams and to constantly monitor the body for the seven major cancer symptoms. Describing education as "the third big front in the war against cancer" (after research and treatment), he urges audiences to learn more about the disease. In particular, the film highlights the role of the WFA: "public meetings arranged by leaders in the war against cancer are being held throughout the country under the auspices of the Women's Field Army of the American Society for the Control of Cancer." The physician concludes, "Cancer is curable when taken in time. To you who say with me, I choose to live, I say remember that early cancer can be cured. Don't take a chance with cancer. Don't waste time with worry. Don't delay."

At last, Brown visits a doctor and explains her concern. The doctor orders a biopsy of Brown's breast tissue, and the viewer finally learns that a breast abnormality is the cause of Brown's anxiety. Describing the pathology lab as a "division of intelligence," the narrator assures the viewer that Brown's diagnosis would be quick and efficient. After being anesthetized for the surgery, Brown remains unconscious, and the pathologists examine her cells. Because some cells in the biopsy are cancerous, "a skilled team of surgeons and nurses swings into action." In a script characteristic of the early 1940s, the surgeons remove Brown's breast without consulting her.[92] The film glosses over the surgery and recovery phase and jumps immediately to her reunion with the family outside of the hospital.

As Brown hugs her family, the narrator speaks: "Mrs. Brown is going home. Her cancer was an early one, and the prompt operation saved her life." The film ignores the effects of mastectomy and the psychological trauma of this operation. The final scene of the film depicts Brown at a WFA recruitment station, enlisting in the Women's Field Army so that she could "educate others to save lives."

The message of prompt attention and medical consultation is obvious in this film. Produced by male associates of the ASCC, in cooperation with the U.S. Public Health Service, the film worked to reinforce the message of early detection, particularly with female audiences.

The film captured the emerging tendency to teach women about cancer by repeating this message in multiple genres. Education had always been a cornerstone of the ASCC, but by the 1930s, when women sponsored films with female cancer patients and hosted educational speakers who stressed early detection, they helped reinforce the message. Hundreds of thousands of women donned military uniforms and endorsed the message of early detection, legitimizing this medical theory for a lay, female audience. By tapping into women's clubs and networks, cancer educators gained access to a culture of reform, where women embraced causes specific to their health and their gender. Although it is impossible to know how audiences responded to these narratives, the frequent repetition of plots that focused on female characters, most of whom were also portrayed as mothers and caretakers of the home, reflected a cultural assumption that the message of early detection would resonate with middle-class female audiences. Authors, filmmakers, and educators (male and female alike) shared these cancer narratives as one way to teach the public about cancer, the risk it posed for women, and the merits of early detection.

Conclusion

One of the few female representatives in Congress in the 1930s, Edith Nourse Rogers, recognized the significant contribution of women in cancer education. Rogers applauded the 1937 passage of the bill that created the National Cancer Institute, but she urged additional support for WFA programs, arguing that financial allocations for cancer research should be complemented by support for cancer awareness movements across the nation. Throughout the 1930s women's clubs offered spaces where the public discussion of cancer could flourish. Women identified breast, cervical, and uterine cancers as diseases peculiar to their sex and informed each other about the value of early detection.

When Florence Becker and Joseph Bloodgood started the ASMF,

they turned to all-female organizations as an audience for cervical cancer information, a subject considered by some as too intimate for mixed audiences. Once the education programs were started, they recruited female volunteers who were willing to spread the message of early detection. The ASMF encouraged women to take responsibility for their health and demand services that medical practitioners might otherwise neglect. This movement differed from the women's health movement today, which insists that laywomen and patients be represented on review committees and challenges the premise of many scientific theories.[93] However, the ASMF suggested the importance of including, consulting with, and educating women when designing health programs for them.

The Sims program offered a model for the Women's Field Army, which emerged a few years later. Both depended on women's clubs to spread their message, used female networks to recruit more volunteers, and articulated concerns for women's health. The WFA differed from the Sims movement in its scope and ambition. Although originally it shared the Sims mission and focus on the high rate of female cancers, particularly cancers of the breast and cervix, over time it addressed broader concerns. The WFA adopted a vision of women as caretakers who would educate men and women about cancer. As National Commander Marjorie Illig explained, "As women I think we may well be proud of the part we are playing in this war to save human life. It is right that women should take the leadership in this fight. After all, we have more cases of cancer than do men. Yet in a deeper sense fighting all diseases is a woman's task. The care of the health, the nursing of the sick, the healing of the injured—these are things which require a woman's patience and a woman's courage."[94]

As WFA cancer awareness efforts increasingly embraced male and family audiences, its messages became simpler, and the women's consciousness evident in the early years lessened. As Illig's comments illustrated, by 1938 the WFA continued to recognize female susceptibility to cancer, but it also prioritized women's role as the caretakers of the nation's health.

3

From Awareness to Screening

EARLY DETECTION REDEFINED

Between 1941 and 1945, U.S. involvement in World War II distracted from some of the advances in cancer control. Many researchers and scientists who were invested in cancer studies shifted their attention to military research, including the creation of the A-bomb. As historian James Patterson has argued, "The war years were discouraging ones for the alliance against cancer."[1] Military enlistment created a shortage of male medical talent and a small pool of researchers. Many women joined the war effort, either by working in manufacturing plants or by shifting voluntary efforts toward war work.[2]

The Women's Field Army (WFA) continued its educational initiatives and fund-raising drives throughout the course of the war, however. It responded to war shortages in various ways, including salvaging initiatives, which converted used materials into surgical supplies. As Ella Rigney, a leader of the New York City WFA claimed, "the battle against the disease must not be slackened because of the immediate demands of the war."[3] Likewise, Representative Edith Nourse Rogers, who had successfully introduced a congressional bill designating April as "cancer control month" in 1938, gave speeches during the war years that stressed the importance of maintaining cancer education programs and postwar planning to expand cancer awareness and services.[4]

The success of science in the war years suggested enormous possibilities for cancer control in the future. Public audiences, medical professionals, and scientists were excited by the prospect of curing cancer. Although the notion of a cancer cure had existed for hundreds of years, it now resonated in a culture of postwar prosperity and scientific accomplishment. The United States had successfully demonstrated that it could divide the atom, and it had harnessed this energy to create the atomic bomb. The nation's sense of power was enhanced by the realization that no other country could match this accomplishment.[5] Moreover, the American public and much of the world witnessed equally spectacular medical discoveries, most notably the mass production of penicillin, which dramatically improved disease outcomes.[6] Within this climate, women and men devoted to cancer education envisioned short-term innovations in medical technology and cancer research that would facilitate cancer screening and treatment.

With this in mind, Mary Lasker, an influential New York philanthropist, businesswoman, and political lobbyist, considered major transformations in the American Society for the Control of Cancer (ASCC). Specifically, she wanted to recreate the society into a powerful organization that prioritized cancer research. Well versed in public relations, connected to the financial center of New York City and political circles in Washington, D.C., networked with important business professionals, and appalled by the limited budget of the largest cancer society in the United States, Lasker played a leading role in the creation of the American Cancer Society (ACS) in the mid-1940s.[7] In spite of notable opposition from medical leaders, between 1943 and 1945 Lasker convinced the ASCC/ACS to change the composition of the board of directors to include more lay members and more experts in financial management. She also encouraged the ACS to earmark one-quarter of its budget for research. This financial reorganization allowed the ACS to sponsor early cancer screening in the 1950s, including the early clinical trials of the vaginal smear.[8] As ACS administrative director Edwin MacEwan wrote to Lasker in 1946, "I learned that you were the person to whom present and potential cancer patients owe everything and that you alone really initiated the rebirth of the American Cancer Society late in 1944."[9]

The Creation of the American Cancer Society

Founded in 1913, the American Society for the Control of Cancer had consistently identified three goals: education, service, and research. Until midcentury, however, and largely due to the limited budget, the society contributed little to cancer research. Instead, the organization focused almost exclusively on cancer awareness and recruited women to teach the merits of early detection followed by surgical treatment. Throughout its history, women had participated in ASCC programs and served as liaisons between the medical professionals and lay female audiences, as demonstrated by the Women's Field Army. The women who were most often recognized publicly by the ASCC tended to be wealthy philanthropists who hosted benefits for the society, but thousands of women routinely assisted the ASCC in its educational efforts. The men who dominated the ASCC tended to be medical professionals, who had created the society to deliver their messages of early detection.[10]

When Mary Lasker inquired about the role and purpose of the ASCC in 1943, she learned that the organization had no money to support research. Somewhat astounded by this discovery, she immediately contemplated ways to reorganize the society.[11] One of the most powerful women in mid-twentieth century New York City, and perhaps the United States, Lasker demonstrated that women could orchestrate changes in male-dominated medical societies. Moreover, she effectively established that the public could influence government appropriations for medical research by employing public relations tools.[12]

Born in Watertown, Wisconsin, in 1900, Mary Lasker's childhood memories included a distinct version of one woman's experience with cancer. At the age of three or four, the family's laundress, Mrs. Belter, had cancer treatment. Lasker learned of the diagnosis

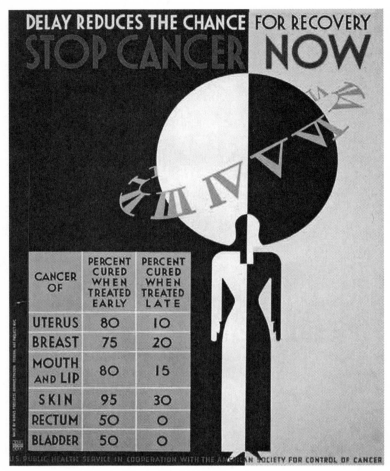

DELAY REDUCES THE CHANCE FOR RECOVERY

STOP CANCER NOW

CANCER OF	PERCENT CURED WHEN TREATED EARLY	PERCENT CURED WHEN TREATED LATE
UTERUS	80	10
BREAST	75	20
MOUTH AND LIP	80	15
SKIN	95	30
RECTUM	50	0
BLADDER	50	0

U.S. PUBLIC HEALTH SERVICE IN COOPERATION WITH THE AMERICAN SOCIETY FOR CONTROL OF CANCER

"Stop Cancer Now." This poster promoted early detection of cancer. It was created by Christopher Denoon in 1938 through the Works Progress Administration. (Library of Congress)

from her mother, who explained, "Mrs. Belter has had cancer and her breasts have been removed." Lasker responded, "What do you mean? Cut off?" When her mother responded affirmatively, Lasker thought, "This shouldn't happen to anybody."[13] Ultimately, Mrs. Belter survived, and the memory encouraged Lasker's belief that cancer

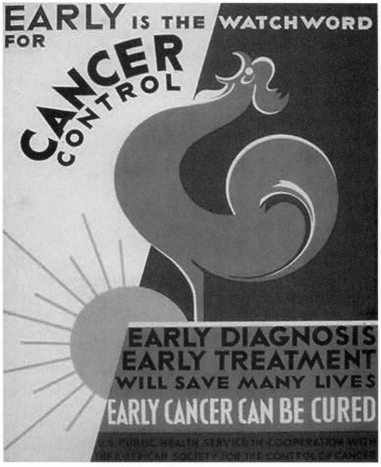

"Early Is the Watchword." This poster taught audiences that early cancer could be cured. It was created by Christopher Denoon in 1938 through the Works Progress Administration. (Library of Congress)

treatment could be effective.[14] In an oral interview conducted in 1976, Lasker still recalled the vividness of her childhood reaction to the disease: "I'll never forget my anger at hearing about this disease that caused such suffering and mutilation and my thinking that something should be done about this."[15]

Another encounter with the devastating effects of cancer, Lasker remembered, occurred in the late 1920s, when Mrs. John Dorr was diagnosed with breast cancer. The mother of one of Lasker's good friends, Mrs. Dorr told Lasker about a lump on her breast while both women were visiting Europe. Lasker encouraged Dorr to visit a physician, and after some delay, and her return to the United States, Dorr did. Convinced of the importance of early detection when she recounted the story, Lasker believed, "It is possible that that short delay may have made the difference between her living and dying. In any case, she died after about two years, really after a great deal of agony. This puzzled and infuriated me, because I found so little had been done in that time about cancer."[16] Two decades later, when Lasker ushered in the transformation of the American Cancer Society, she would mention these early memories that had inspired her to engage in cancer work.

Privileged in many regards, Lasker traveled internationally at a young age, attended boarding school at Milwaukee Downer Seminary, and completed two years at the University of Wisconsin before leaving Wisconsin for health issues related to fatigue and anemia. Three years later, she completed her undergraduate degree at Radcliffe, graduating cum laude. After graduation, she traveled throughout Europe, to France, Italy, and England. On New Year's Eve, 1923, she met art dealer Paul Reinhardt and began working in his galleries the next year. In 1925 she agreed to marry Reinhardt if he stopped drinking for one year.[17] They wed in May 1926.

An astute financier and art dealer, Lasker invested wisely in the early years of her marriage. She purchased a Modigliani for $300 and a Matisse for $600 and began investing in stock in 1926. Soon before the stock market crash of 1929, she sold her stock in order to purchase additional art. Although Reinhardt had kept his promise of sobriety for years, in 1930 he began drinking again; and by 1934 Mary Lasker had divorced him and established herself as an independent and successful businesswoman.

In the 1930s Mary Lasker extended her business interests and engaged in industrial design work. She also cultivated friendships with influential people throughout the nation. As one example, the guest list of one evening party she hosted included such luminaries as birth control advocate Margaret Sanger and First Lady Eleanor Roosevelt. In 1940, when she met and later married advertising executive Albert Lasker, her social, political, and business connections expanded even more broadly.

Mary Lasker pursued an interest in health issues throughout the 1930s. She supported birth control efforts and expressed concern about financing for health care and health insurance coverage. In late 1939, when Lasker's maid was diagnosed with cancer, Lasker shifted her attention to cancer, learning about the dearth of information and services provided by the American Society for the Control of Cancer. This experience, combined with her memories of other women who had struggled with cancer, pushed her to learn more about the cancer problem. Fueled by memories of her laundress, frustrated with the suffering caused by cancer, and convinced that the ASCC needed to fund research, Lasker investigated the status of the ASCC, cancer research, political support for cancer, and more.[18]

By 1943, when Mary Lasker considered transforming the ASCC, she was married to her second husband, Albert Lasker. A public relations expert who had earned a national reputation for his work, he sold his firm Lord & Thomas in 1942. The firm was renamed Foote, Cone & Belding, in recognition of the vice presidents who bought it. Renowned for his public relations campaigns for such clients as Sunkist, Kleenex, Kotex, and Lucky Strike (advertisements that encouraged cigarettes for women), Albert Lasker had amassed a small fortune from his success.[19] Mary Lasker also had resources of her own, including her valuable art collection. Wealthy, socially connected, and committed to cancer control, Mary Lasker envisioned a new business model for the ASCC. When she read about the New York City Cancer Committee campaign to raise $500,000 for cancer research, she could not believe the size of the budget. "In business," she summarized, "$500,000 wouldn't even be a suitable sum to use for an advertising campaign for a toothpaste."[20]

As one indication of Mary Lasker's clout, once she decided to become involved with the cancer problem, she immediately contacted ASCC executive director C. C. Little, who agreed to meet her. On November 22, 1943, Lasker and Little met at the ASCC office on Madison Avenue. Lasker inquired about the society's budget, its program, and its financial needs. Eager to publish his book, *Cancer: A Study for Laymen*, Little admitted the limited financial resources of the organization. He requested $4,000 to publish this book and an additional $1,000 for meetings with doctors and science writers. Lasker agreed to this sum and secured $5,000 for the ASCC.[21]

These conversations revealed that the society had few funds for research. As Lasker commiserated with her friend and fellow health activist Florence Mahoney after the meeting, "They weren't going to eliminate cancer; they were just going to 'control' it, but they were going to control it without any research as they raised no money for research at all." Lasker was equally critical of the educational agenda of the ASCC and the impact of women in the WFA. Although she supported education, she believed that more attention needed to be directed to the prevention of cancer and its cure. In addition, she believed the WFA was a "well-intentioned" group but ineffectual at raising large amounts of money for much-needed research funds.[22]

At this initial meeting between Mary Lasker and Little, Little asked if Albert Lasker might be willing to serve as chair of a public relations committee for the ASCC. Mary Lasker mentioned her husband's poor health but promised to introduce Little to public relations expert Emerson Foote. She arranged a meeting between the two within a month. Mary Lasker's access to professional contacts would immediately improve the public profile of the ASCC. Foote brought professional public relations experience to the organization. In addition, he was inspired to engage in cancer work after losing both of his parents to the disease.[23]

Lasker also reviewed literature on the disease and contemporary cancer research. In 1943 she requested reports from the National Cancer Institute, and she collected information about research funding sources, lamenting the limited support from the federal government and the ASCC.[24] Her personal papers contain multiple publications from the 1940s about the state of cancer research, which ranged from reprints of medical journals to copies of popular articles in women's magazines, such as "Killer of Women" from a 1947 *Ladies' Home Journal*.[25]

Lasker challenged the parochial nature of the ASCC, which tended to focus on education at the expense of medical research. Although the organization nodded its head to research in its mission statement, Lasker quickly surmised that it offered little financial support to research initiatives. She envisioned a cancer society that could inform patients and physicians, support research, and offer services to patients. In 1944 she began listing hundreds of prominent individuals who might support such a cancer society and outlined a new organizational structure for the ASCC. In this diagram a board of directors would include lay professionals, and the board would oversee groups that focused on major initiatives such as fund-raising, research, and public relations. Less than a year later, Lasker described the reorganization as one that led to the creation of a "comprehensive attack on cancer." The new society would have, in addition to the reorganized board of directors, a separate board of medical directors, a long-term research agenda, and a plan that offered services to patients. Similar to Elise Mead's work in collecting dues after the creation of the ASCC, Lasker facilitated the creation of different types of membership, ranging from a lifetime membership for $100 to annual dues of $5.[26]

Undeterred by opposition from medical professionals who wanted to retain the original composition of the board (a majority of M.D.s and a handful of lay professionals), Lasker insisted that medical experts should not run the organization. "They'd been in the business for 36 years," she pointed out, "and had not raised a cent for research."[27] She questioned the capabilities of medical doctors in the fields of business relations, fund-raising, and publicity. By 1944 she had convinced the society that Emerson Foote should have a seat on the board of directors and that the society should hire a full-time public relations officer (half of whose salary was paid for by Foote, Cone & Belding). In addition, Lewis Douglas (Mutual Life), Elmer Bobst (pharmaceuticals), and Thomas Braniff (Braniff Airways) joined the board within a few years.[28]

After altering the composition of the board of directors, Mary Lasker decided to boost fund-raising for the cancer society. In a 1944 meeting with a leading ASCC supporter, Dr. Cornelius Rhoads, and public relations expert Emerson Foote, Lasker explicitly suggested that she would help the society raise money for research if the society would recognize research as a top priority. Following this meeting, Lasker secured $2,400 for research, informing the society, "This gift which was solicited on the basis that the Cancer Society intends to create such a Research Fund and small Research Committee, is, I hope, the first of many that will come to the society in the future." In case her inferences were missed, she included an address for the return of the money if the ASCC did not comply with her wishes to further cancer research.[29]

In July 1944 Lasker pushed her public relations and fund-raising campaign further ahead. During lunch with an editor of *Reader's Digest*, Mrs. James Monahan, who worked under the pseudonym Lois Mattox Miller, Lasker discussed the devastating statistics about modern cancer and late detection.[30] Lasker suggested that Mattox Miller include an article about cancer in her popular magazine, with a simple byline that read that any donations could be sent to the society. As Mattox Miller wrote, "In this case, we could point out the need for funds, educational work, frequent examinations, and all the other points that would be helpful in controlling cancer."[31] Mattox Miller obliged Lasker, and between October 1944 and April 1945 three articles appeared in *Reader's Digest* with a tagline that requested financial contributions. As a result, readers sent the society over $60,000. Two additional articles brought the total to over $130,000.[32] Although a small initiative, these two women demonstrated how mass appeals could generate funds for research.

In a final gesture that marked the formal reorganization of the ASCC, Lasker met with Foote to explain that she found the name of the society "very cumbersome." Foote subsequently urged the board to consider a name change, and by the fall of 1944 the board had adopted the new name, the American Cancer Society. Within three years, Lasker had transformed the ASCC into a national philanthropic organization that supported major research projects. Although invited to join the board, Mary Lasker declined in favor of her husband, Albert Lasker. Committed to the professionalization of the board and its inclusion of public relations experts, it seems that Lasker prioritized her husband's social and political clout as important to the newly created ACS. She also conformed to dominant gender norms that privileged male experience and expertise on executive committees. The newly elected board of directors included a dozen new members, all male, and many who also served as presidents of leading U.S. companies, with experience in marketing and public relations. However, Mary Lasker continued to work behind the scenes and in ways that maximized her influence.[33] As she had anticipated with the reorganization, in an era when the prospect for a cancer cure seemed certain, the public could be persuaded to donate money for cancer research.[34]

Albert Lasker joined Mary Lasker's efforts to raise cancer funds. In 1944 he successfully solicited a contribution of $50,000 from Lever Brothers. Moreover, he helped the organization raise $4 million in 1945, and he became increasingly invested in cancer research.[35] He accepted a nomination to the board of directors of the ACS in May 1945. Mary Lasker continued to agitate for research funds but resisted any formal association with the ACS until the 1950s. As she explained it, "I'm always best on the outside."[36]

The newly formed American Cancer Society articulated a mission that explicitly identified research funding as its primary goal. It benefited from popular culture that supported scientific research. As explained in *Women's Home Companion*, "World War II taught one lesson of incalculable importance. The lesson: that with unlimited money to spend we can buy the answers to almost any scientific problem."[37] Cancer educators capitalized on the emerging faith in science to encourage support for early detection programs and research programs.

Early efforts to increase financial contributions to the ACS proved successful. Beginning with the *Reader's Digest* columns, thousands of readers sent in contributions that would ensure research funding. The reconfiguration of board members promised large financial contributions as well. By late 1944, the American Cancer Society had become the principal nongovernmental funding agency for cancer research in the country. In its first year, it directed $1 million of its $4 million in revenue to research. As historian James Patterson has surmised, "In the minds of many Americans the conquest of cancer was the next great challenge—to be met in the same manner that the physicists had taken on the mysteries of the atom."[38]

Cancer Education: Narratives and Technology

The ACS's new emphasis on securing research funds did not distract from the traditional educational agenda of the ASCC. Education campaigns of the mid-twentieth century continued to stress the importance of early detection while working to convince Americans that cancer research funding was an equally important goal. Magazine articles, posters, films, and educational pamphlets presented cancer as a threatening disease, but one that could be controlled with adequate funds and education. Awareness campaigns still frequently addressed women and increasingly relied on foil characters who did or did not comply with ACS guidelines to emphasize the importance of early detection. These cancer narratives explicitly outlined "good" and "bad" behavior for female patients.

A pharmaceutical advertisement in *Hygeia*, a leading popular health magazine, epitomized this trend. This full-page 1945 advertisement depicted two women side by side, each within a frame. The accompanying text explained that the woman was either "wise" or "foolish" about her health care. The "wise" woman noticed a lump in her breast, immediately consulted a physician, received treatment, and survived. This woman was portrayed as happy and healthy, without any indications that she has or had cancer. Her physical surroundings suggest domestic bliss. Presumably a mother, she sews and observes her two children who play nearby. The neighboring picture featured a "foolish" woman who ignored the lump in her breast. By the time she had the operation, it "showed nothing could be done as disease had spread too far." This woman is shown alone in a hospital room without familial support. Shadowed in dark tones, thin, apparently depressed, and presumably dying, the message resonated loudly. Women were responsible for detecting cancer in its early stages, and failure to do so had dire consequences.[39]

This advertisement reflected a common theme in postwar literature and rhetoric about female cancers and early detection. Echoing messages introduced in the first decades of the century, it implied that a woman's willingness to follow simple steps of early detection would determine whether she would survive. Educational campaigns never undermined the power of the physician to cure the disease and instead placed the burden of detection on individual behavior. Campaigns offered a generic definition of cancer based on the notion of a localized growth that could be surgically excised in early stages. In this definition cancer could be controlled, and variances due to cancer types, severity, or degree were ignored. Therefore, women's behavior became the key variable in cancer control. Put more bluntly, if a woman with cancer failed to follow early detection principles, death seemed inevitable, and the victim assumed the blame.

Popular cancer literature rarely recognized the multifaceted nature of a cancer diagnosis that started with detection of symptoms but then might include physician visits, surgical biopsy, and a variety of options for surgical treatment, radiation, and after World War II even chemotherapy.[40] In this instance, the advertisement referred to an "operation," but it failed to describe the procedure and said nothing about breast excision or mastectomy. One can assume that the "wise" women had a mastectomy, but judging from her appearance she wore a prosthesis that disguised it. These messages made no references to losing a breast, the nature of aggressive cancers that could not be cured by surgery, the reality of unsuccessful treatment, or the rate of metastasis.

This reactionary strategy was dependent on the assumption that

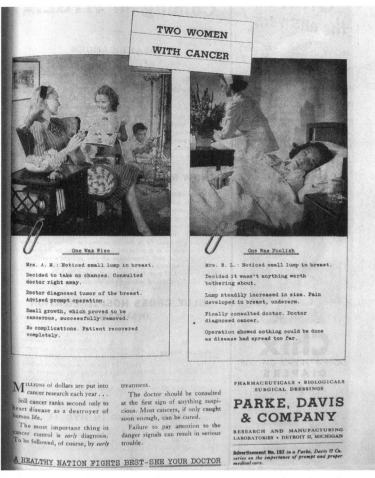

Parke, Davis, and Company advertisement promoting the value of cancer awareness, placed in popular periodicals, including *Hygeia*, in 1945. (Courtesy of Pfizer)

women had learned the basic instructions regarding cancer symptoms and that physicians could treat the disease. The narratives further implied that women must not react poorly to potential cancer symptoms. "The patient herself is the first line of defense against cancer," another 1945 *Hygeia* article noted. "It is her responsibility to watch for those signs of cancer which can be seen or felt by her, to consult a competent physician *immediately* if she notes a cancer sign or symptom, and, whether she has evidence of the disease or not, to present herself to her physician regularly for a thorough physical examination." In case that message was not clear enough, the article reiterated, "The exterior of the body, of course, is easily inspected and examined by the patient herself and the responsibility for detecting the earliest signs of external cancer therefore is on her. If she does not watch for those signs, or if, after discovering them, she does not seek competent medical care until cancer has passed its early, most curable stage, she has no one to blame for the consequences but herself."[41]

Prioritizing early detection as the most significant factor in avoiding death from cancer and associating this outcome with terms such as "easy" suggested that the ability to survive cancer lay within each woman's power. Moreover, the rhetoric of early detection placed a burden on women to detect cancer, implicitly blamed women for late-stage diagnoses, and exaggerated the obvious nature of cancer symptoms. Frequent claims that any "wide-awake," "alert," or "wise" woman would recognize cancer painted women who did not notice early cancer symptoms as "modest," "ashamed," or "foolish." These generalizations ignored the difficulty of early detection, such as lumps that were too small to feel, and the prohibitive costs of medical consultation. The popular education campaign, although created and promulgated by women, tended to rely on gendered assumptions about female modesty and to reinforce the idea that women needed to change their behavior and overcome shame about their bodies for treatment to become truly effective.[42] Finally, the assumption that doctors could cure cancer in its earliest phases further valorized a profession that was already highly esteemed in postwar culture.[43] Although women participating in cancer awareness effectively conveyed the importance of early detection, they did little to challenge the gender and medical norms of the mid-twentieth century.

A second literary tool often applied in the postwar era was a growing reliance on autobiographical narratives for cancer education.

Articles such as "I Had Cancer" and "Cancer—I've Had It" used the first-person point of view to convey the relevance of cancer detection to readers' lives. Published in popular women's magazines, these articles mirrored earlier educational efforts and reinforced the notion that early detection promised survival while delayed detection might result in death.[44]

In early 1947 *Ladies' Home Journal* published Marion Flexner's autobiographical story about breast cancer, in which she stressed the importance of her early diagnosis. Despite the class- and race-specific nature of this story (Flexner was a wealthy white woman), it offered a blunt and enlightened discussion of cancer, diagnosis, and treatment. Flexner's husband, who was also her physician, explained that he would treat her cancerous lump with a radical mastectomy. This unusual physician-patient relationship provided an intimate example of the value of responding to cancer symptoms quickly. As readers inferred, no husband would needlessly operate on his wife. The article served to convince readers that they needed to trust their physician and believe that he or she was acting in the patient's best interest.[45]

Flexner relied on autobiography to share the details of her cancer diagnosis. In particular, she described the unsettling discovery of a lump in her breast while putting on a brassiere. She described the recommended treatment, a radical mastectomy, and revealed her postoperative concerns, including her anxiety over the breast prosthesis.[46]

In the convention of celebrating early detection and physicians, Flexner stressed that early detection had ensured her survival. Moreover, the doctor/husband played the role of a stable and authoritative male healer. As he pointed out, "There is no such thing as a *little* cancer. But, we know that if cancer is removed early enough—and yours was the second smallest I've ever seen—the great majority of patients will make a complete recovery." Typical of midcentury popular cancer literature, the article conflated theories of controlling cancer, curing cancer, and treating the disease. The final line of the article recounted the parting words of her husband/physician, "I think you're cured."[47]

A month later, the *Ladies' Home Journal* published another biography about breast cancer. Mary Roberts Rinehart, one of the most successful detective-story writers of the twentieth century, allowed Gretta Palmer to write a story about Rinehart's cancer experience.[48] Palmer wrote the profile, "I Had Cancer," in 1947, eleven years after Rinehart's diagnosis.[49] The eleven-year window between Rinehart's diagnosis and her willingness to share her story with a broad audience may suggest that the postwar trends fostered new space for cancer narratives and a greater willingness among women to make their stories known. The article chronicled Rinehart's literary success, stressed her devotion to her family, and recognized her "wisdom" that proved critical to surviving cancer. As Rinehart summarized, "No. There is nothing for the modern woman to fear about most cases of cancer. Nothing except delay!"[50]

Once again, this article emphasized that delayed diagnosis might lead to death, while early detection saved lives. For example, the reader learned that Rinehart lost a daughter-in-law who "tragically enough, suspected that she was a victim of cancer, but told no one and paid the ultimate price for her secret."[51] Rinehart shared her story with millions of readers because she believed that if all women realized that early detection saved lives, fewer women would die from cancer. "This, of all diseases, is one whose course should be clearly understood by all of us," she noted, "for there are few maladies in which neglect, in the early stages, can cost the patient so high a price in hope for recovery." ACS figures supported this claim by stating that women had greater than an 80 percent chance of surviving of early breast cancer cases versus a 40 to 50 percent survival rate for "moderately advanced cases." Often, articles on breast cancer also included taglines about reproductive cancers and early detection.[52]

Although the ACS had reconfigured itself by midcentury, the legacy of the ASCC and its emphasis on early detection continued, especially for women. Women learned that they had a responsibility to respond to cancer symptoms in order for cures to be effective. These messages were repeated in biographical narratives, as well as in illness narratives with foil characters. The familiar use of female characters, references to breast and uterine cancers, and publication in women's magazines advanced the notion that cancer was a female concern. Although the forum for discussions of cancer had broadened, the focus remained rooted in individual behavior. Women promoting cancer awareness continually reinforced this message, teaching individual women about their role in detection. Although this strategy was surely meant to relieve the anxiety and fear associated with the disease, it perpetuated the notion that female cancer was an individual concern versus a community concern. Literary foils and personal narratives were useful devices for stressing early detection, but they would not inspire a communal response from women or any political manifestos about accountability for high breast and cervical cancer rates in the midcentury United States.

Breast Self-Examination

The priority placed on early detection led to innovative trends in breast cancer awareness. Notions of self-examinations had surfaced for decades in vague references to the discovery of a lump while dressing or showering, in instructions about examining the breast for indications of abnormalities, and in assumptions that women would notice disfigurement and lumps in the breast. Until the late 1940s, however, the ACS and its affiliated women's clubs did not offer formal or standardized instruction for breast self-examination (BSE). Not until 1948 did a formal and national program for BSE instruction begin under the sponsorship of the ACS.

In the late 1930s Alfred Popma, a radiologist in Boise, Idaho, began working closely with the ASCC and cancer educators to advocate a program that would encourage women to perform routine breast self-examinations. The first qualified radiologist in the Boise area, Popma served as the director of the Radiology Department at St. Luke's Hospital until 1966. Frequently treating cancer patients and active in the ASCC, Popma participated in statewide cancer awareness initiatives.[53]

When Popma delivered cancer awareness lectures, he often noticed that women desired specific instructions for detecting breast cancer. He therefore decided to formalize detection instruction with a slide show. By 1946, he offered audiences formal BSE instruction, accompanied by visual images of the exam. After receiving profuse praise from audiences for the slide show, Popma produced a sixteen-millimeter film that would demonstrate the most effective way to detect breast lumps.[54]

Unlike earlier educational films produced by the national ACS and informed by its doctrine of the seven major warning signs, Popma's film focused on a single task, the breast self-examination. It did not use drama or narrative to convey its point but instead documented several women performing the exam. A local production, the film was a direct response to the demands of women in Idaho who wanted more instruction on BSE.

Life Saving Fingers featured Popma, an authoritative medical professional, as the narrator. It opened with several familiar messages: early breast cancer could be cured; a painless lump in the breast might be an indication of cancer; a woman needed to discover any lumps in her breast; and only a doctor could definitely diagnose cancer. The film urged women to familiarize themselves with the normal feel of breast tissue in order to recognize any abnormalities in the tissue. Finally, it recommended regular, even daily, breast self-examinations. The 1948 short film, produced by the Idaho chapter of the ACS, featured a woman, naked from waist upward, who meticulously performed the breast self-examination.[55]

Very factual in tone and straightforward in its instruction, the film shows the primary female character sitting before a mirror with her breasts exposed. Because no breast self-examination film had ever been produced, this film became one of the first cancer awareness films to dismiss notions of propriety and visually depict the examination. The narrator reminds the viewer to follow simple steps of examining the normal shape of her breasts, raising and lowering her arms to search for abnormalities, and to note any peculiarities, such as lopsided breasts. Popma suggests a woman use her right hand to examine her left breast, and vice versa. As he explains, "Do not pinch. Use only the tips of the fingers, pressing gently but firmly on the breast tissue. Beginning at the inner part of the breast, roll the tissue gently, with the fingertips compressing the breast against the chest wall. You will often be able to feel the ribs through the breast tissue."

The female character performs her BSE while staring into the lens of the camera. Imagining the camera lens as a mirror, the viewer gained a glimpse of the process from this useful perspective. The narrator reminds the viewer to be patient, examine the entire breast, and work the fingers gradually toward the armpit. Another image shows how fingers could be moved in small circles to better feel the breast tissue. The narrator recommends that a woman examine her nipple by "gently compressing the tissue immediately surrounding the nipple between the thumb and first finger," again reminding the viewer not to pinch. *Life Saving Fingers* then features three additional female characters, all middle-aged white women, who also perform breast self-examinations. It uses animation to detail the common locations of breast cancer and identifies the common areas for metastases— the armpit and collarbone. *Life Saving Fingers* concludes by telling all viewers to perform self-examinations regularly and to direct any suspicions of cancer to a physician for a diagnosis.

The primary female actor in this film volunteered for the role in order to promote breast cancer education. Her mother had recently died from breast cancer and the woman wanted to contribute to this innovative cancer awareness project. She volunteered to expose her breasts in front of the camera as a way to help others. A grassroots project, the film was shot inside Popma's home, and also featured a nurse and three additional female volunteers. The twenty-one-minute film on the breast self-examination was the first of its kind.[56]

The film generated a positive response, indicating that women wanted this instruction. Audiences commented on its usefulness, and within a few years the local production gained national distribution status. Reiterating the importance of medical expertise in cancer awareness programming, the Idaho ACS distributed copies of the film in canisters with a capitalized and underlined warning, "TO BE

SHOWN ONLY WITH A MEDICAL SPEAKER PRESENT." The Idaho chapter wanted to demonstrate that it was neither challenging medical opinion nor suggesting that a film could replace the voice of a medical specialist. It insisted that each viewing of the film be followed by a question-and-answer session with a medical specialist. The presence of a medical professional lent the film a greater sense of authority and helped ensure that the ACS would continue to cooperate with the medical profession as it ventured into educational films of the BSE.[57]

The label pasted to each film canister of *Life Saving Fingers* reminds us of the hierarchy that existed between female educators who advanced cancer awareness and the medical professionals who lectured on cancer control. In Idaho, and throughout the United States, physicians were recognized as more knowledgeable, powerful, and authoritative than any female volunteers. As men asserted their professional expertise, however, women persisted in advancing the educational agenda. Convinced by the merits of early detection, women working for the ACS continued to network and inform female communities about cancer risks. Although they never challenged cancer policy, they actively supported the theory of early detection and self-examination by continually participating in cancer awareness programming.

A year later, in 1949, the American Cancer Society and the National Cancer Institute cooperated in the production of a second film that addressed breast self-examination. Produced specifically for "medical and allied professionals," *Cancer: The Problem of Early Diagnosis* offered an overview of five types of cancer: breast, cervical, stomach, rectal, and lung cancers. Targeting a far different audience than Popma's film, *Cancer* defined breast cancer as a "grave health problem of our time." Furthermore, it acknowledged medical difficulties facing the profession, including the subtle and often uncertain distinctions between the diagnosis of abnormal breasts without disease, with benign disease, and with malignant disease. Admitting that physicians could offer only imperfect physical diagnosis, the film emphasized, "Only by a microscopic examination of tissue specimens can a diagnosis of breast cancer be made with scientific accuracy." It urged physicians to learn about the clinical symptoms of breast cancer and to treat breast cancer aggressively, but it also exposed the limits of the medical profession. Films produced for popular audiences erased the uncertainty evident in this production, which would only be viewed by those "within" the profession.[58]

Cancer offered a sophisticated discussion of the disease. First, it traced the clinical pathology of cancer, identifying the earliest manifestation of cancer as a lump in the breast that could be detected by palpation or "finger manipulation." The film featured pictures of four women with visible breast irregularities, including one image of a woman whose breast had been amputated. Then, in a series of approximately eight images, the film depicted breast deformities that ranged from subtle indications of cancer, such as a slight dimple in the breast, to images of advanced and untreated breast cancer. Many of these images included disfigurement and exposed the deformity that cancer could cause. The film stressed the value of a visual and physical examination but consistently warned that biopsy offered the only accurate diagnostic tool. A discussion of Paget's disease, indicated by sores on the nipple, followed.[59]

Unlike popular films, this film stressed the ambiguity of a clinical breast examination. Whereas films for laywomen insisted that breast cancer could be detected simply, films for professionals admitted that clinical manifestations might be difficult to determine. Popular films taught women that cancer could be cured, yet this medical film featured vivid depictions of cancerous breasts that illustrated the destructive nature of the disease. In the same vein that Popma reminded women to be "patient," this narrator urged the medical profession to conduct "painstaking" breast examinations twice a year.

Unlike *Life Saving Fingers*, which offered women a model for conducting a breast self-examination, *Cancer* described a clinical breast examination in three parts. First, it encouraged practitioners to conduct a visual examination, which might reveal suspicious changes in the size, shape, contour, and skin of the breast. Second, it explained that light examinations could reveal lumps/density in the breasts by directing rays through the breast tissue and studying the shadow this produced. Third, palpating the breast and squeezing the nipples might reveal breast irregularities: "the practitioner is truly seeing with his fingers, employing the single most important clinical diagnostic method for discovery of early breast cancer." The examinations, each demonstrated by a physician and patient in the film, stressed the need for a methodical approach that divided the breast into quadrants or regions.[60]

Unlike popular educational material, which rarely dealt with metastasis, this medical film bluntly stated that if cancer had spread to the axillary nodes, the patient's chance of survival was poor. Moreover, it reiterated the conventional cancer treatment protocol of the twentieth century, telling practitioners that treatment must be prompt, that biopsy offered accurate diagnosis, and that the most effective treatment was radical surgery. "Except in low [few] instances, a simple mastectomy has no place in the management of breast cancer," the film advised. Finally, the film promoted postoperative care and pictured a woman who had a mastectomy performing arm exercises after her surgery.

The film ended on a positive but cautionary note that repeated the importance of radical surgery: "Breast cancer is a curable disease. Clinical proof attests to the benefits of radical mastectomy." It asked doctors to engage in popular education and inform women about the importance of regular breast self-examinations. Furthermore, it reminded physicians to spread this message throughout the profession so that doctors, too, would recognize the value of this periodic examination. "Only the physician's high index of early suspicion followed at once by an accurate diagnosis makes possible the effective treatment of the cancer patient," the film concluded.

Although the three main themes of this film—early detection, accurate diagnosis, and effective treatment—also permeated the popular awareness campaign, this medical film introduced additional dimensions of the disease that were deliberately excluded from programs for lay audiences. Specifically, it included explicit and disturbing images of cancer that underscored the invasive nature of the disease. Also, it discussed radical mastectomy and documented the effects of breast amputation. Finally, it recognized the high rate of recurrence, the likelihood and danger of metastasis, and the difficulty of early detection. *Cancer* acknowledged the importance of teaching breast self-examination to female patients, yet it failed to explore the best way to educate patients. Notably vague about this procedural step, the film reflected the assumption that while medical experts focused on science, nonspecialists could focus on education. This patronizing attitude relegated women to a less influential role in midcentury cancer control.

In the following year the ACS, the National Cancer Institute, and the U.S. Public Health Service cooperated in producing *Breast Self-Examination: A Film for Women's Groups on Breast Cancer*.[61] Designed for a broad female viewership, this film again highlighted the value of early detection. In an opening scene that mirrors the women's club meeting in the earlier film *Choose To Live*, the camera scans a meeting of white, middle- and upper-class women clad in hats discussing how "each of us can do something to protect ourselves against this disease, a motif that once again stressed the role of individual compliance in cancer control. A sign at the door reads, "Central Women's Health Lecture by Sutton A. Williams, M.D. 2:00 P.M." The dialogue begins rather awkwardly after the lecture ends. A woman invites the audience to ask questions, but a moment of silence ensues. She then admits, "Oh I know some of us may feel reluctant to ask questions about breast cancer, but after all, the only way the doctors have been able to help us is to open up this entire subject to honest and intelligent discussion."[62]

One woman named Mrs. Wright asks Dr. Williams how to perform a breast self-examination, and he advises her to visit her doctor and ask about the technique.[63] Wright follows this advice, and in the next film sequence she learns how to perform a BSE. Obviously, the viewer also learns from this visual demonstration. The doctor deliberately explains every step of the examination as he touches different parts of the breast. He does not press hard, especially compared to contemporary standards. He then shows Wright how to repeat the examination herself and encourages her to do it once a month after her menstrual cycle. The doctor insists that Wright use common sense and not "think too much about it, because thinking too much about cancer isn't healthy for any of us."[64] The physician thus trivializes Wright's concern about cancer, presents the BSE as a powerful and simple tool, and utilizes the model of individual behavior that female educators had instilled throughout the 1930s. The film then follows Wright home, where she repeats the examination in front of a mirror. Moving the examination into the domestic realm bolstered the notion that women were responsible for performing breast self-examinations. Simultaneously, it reinforced gender norms that commonly portrayed women in domestic settings.

Taking its lead from *Life Saving Fingers*, this film also featured women nude from the waist up. In order to gauge audience reaction, the ACS distributed the film selectively. The film premiered at the annual meeting of the American Medical Association in 1950. Throughout the summer it was shown to local, regional, and national medical groups. Finally, select women, such as the presidents of various women's organizations, viewed the film. Once it had met with the approval of these groups, the film was widely distributed. This simple screening process laid bare the patriarchy of the ACS. Women composed the lowest tier of film critics and were only granted access to view the film after it had passed predominantly male medical censors. In spite of their marginalization from health policy related to cancer, women continued to serve as liaisons between the medical profession and large audiences of laywomen, ensuring that educational events would be well attended and cancer philanthropy would continue.

The producers further conveyed the hierarchy and patriarchy of the ACS by opening the film with an announcement that the medical profession had endorsed the film. They proudly defined the final version of the film as one that described breast cancer with "textbook detachment." Reviews confirmed this appraisal. In a positive review of the film, the popular news magazine *Newsweek* described it as "unemotional." Likewise, the specialized medical *Journal of the American Medical Association* claimed the film was "concise and sensible." Unwilling to address the emotional reactions to breast cancer or confront the ways that a diagnosis might change women's lives, the film focused exclusively on breast self-examinations.[65]

Within the first four years of its release, over 5 million women watched the film that depicted the breast self-examination as a "modern" and "powerful" innovation.[66] *Science News Letter* proclaimed, "A NEW and very personal way in which American women can actively fight cancer has been devised. It consists of a motion picture film designed to show them how to examine their own breasts each month for early signs of cancer."[67]

These three films offer a visual reminder that a public discussion of breast cancer existed in many parts of the United States by midcentury. The millions of women eager to see these films attest to the success of cancer awareness efforts that targeted women. Women had successfully created space for cancer education in American culture. Female cancer activists ensured that dozens of women would congregate in a central space, learn about cancer, and participate in question-and-answer sessions about the disease. Women fostered a sense of concern among female populations and responded to that concern with well-orchestrated education initiatives. Women continued to arrange educational programs that served their community, on a local level.

Peggy Lombardo, an ACS volunteer, recounted her efforts to attract a large audience for *Breast Self-Examination* in Jacksonville, Florida. Lombardo started showing the film to small groups of women from women's clubs and churches in 1951. Responding to the audiences' enthusiasm, as well as to multiple requests for additional viewings, Lombardo approached the owner of a local movie theater, Sam Wolfson, and asked him to donate theater space for a public showing of the film. Wolfson agreed. Lombardo then recruited support throughout the community. Local radio stations and newspapers advertised the upcoming film. The Film Projector's Union volunteered time and equipment to run the sixteen-millimeter film. Women's clubs advertised the event and nursing associations encouraged the medical community to attend. The ACS provided childcare and arranged for several doctors to participate in a question-and-answer session after the film. Lombardo described the community's response to the film:

> The morning of the showing was cloudy and rainy and my heart sank when I thought of all those I approached and their willingness to help me and then just have a few in attendance—When I arrived at the theater an hour before the showing and to my joy, there were two lines women waiting to get in—one from each direction and around the block. The showing was a success—so we continued publicity and held it again the following day to another packed theater.
>
> Finally we had requests from women who worked during the day and were unable to attend and requested an evening showing which we held at the YWCA [Young Women's Christian Association]. The executive director of the Florida division of the ACS reported the success of the film in Jacksonville to national—who produced large enough films that could be shown from the theater projection booth and it offered them to all division and units throughout the country on a loan basis.[68]

The success of the film spoke to women's desires to learn the proper technique of the BSE and the pervasiveness of the early detection rhetoric in the postwar era. Moreover, the film's success heralded the increased public discussions of the disease, as awareness programs that once seemed reserved for popular literature, private discussions, or the halls of women's clubs could be found in public arenas.[69] The film clearly targeted an audience reflected by the women depicted in the film. However, in part due to the prompting of leaders such as Lombardo, the film and its message reached a broader audience. Some of the less traditional venues that showed the film included industrial sites, department stores, insurance offices, community centers, housing projects, public libraries, and churches. In Portland, Oregon, a concerted effort to show the film to working women included viewings in canneries, laundries, and union meetings.[70]

This effort to teach women the breast self-examination rested in part on a philosophy that included self-empowerment. As the article "You Can Escape Breast Cancer" preached, "A woman can discover a small lump in her breast that most doctors would miss." The movement taught women to examine their breasts monthly, between menstrual cycles, and to visit a doctor immediately at any sign of irregularity. This article stated as a matter of fact that "there is no place in this perfectly normal procedure for fear, panic, or neurotic obsession."[71] Another article, entitled "How to Prevent 100,000 Cancer Deaths a Year," encouraged women to ask their physicians for regular medical examinations. A community case study that promoted early detection demonstrated, this article contended, that "cancer fear has been replaced with knowledge; terror, by optimism."[72] For some women, the education campaign offered instruction about the breast self-examination and assurance that it was the proper technique to use, and perhaps it lessened their trepidation about the disease. With the breast self-examination, the *Ladies' Home Journal* argued, "every woman has in her own hands the strongest defense known today against a dreaded enemy."[73]

George Papanicolaou and the Vaginal Smear

The perceived success of *The Breast Self-Examination* propelled the ACS to produce a similar film on cervical cancer approximately a decade later, called *Time and Two Women* (1957). Like the effort to teach women about the value of breast self-examinations, the uterine cancer awareness campaign also emphasized the value of early detection.[74] But in midcentury the campaign incorporated contemporary notions of cancer screening technology.[75]

The history of the vaginal smear offers one illustration of the technological innovations that redefined female cancers in the second half of the twentieth century. As scientists, practitioners, female patients, and cancer activists sought ways to detect cancer as early as possible, screening technology gained impressive financial and academic support that shaped cancer awareness advocacy. Undoubtedly, Mary Lasker's influence and emphasis on funding cancer research contributed to the promotion of the Pap smear in U.S. culture. Although cancer educators waited until the late 1950s to launch a cervical cancer screening awareness campaign, the evolution of the technology and the scientific responses to cancer screening dated back to the early twentieth century.

In 1917 George Papanicolaou (1883–1962), a Greek physician, published research in cytology that proved he could trace various stages of the estrous cycle in female guinea pigs.[76] Throughout the next decade he repeated these studies on human specimens (via vaginal discharges obtained from the cervix of the uterus) in an effort to trace cyclical changes. Relying on daily vaginal smears that he obtained from his wife, and later expanding the study to include nurses and patients at the Women's Hospital of the City of New York, Papanicolaou discovered a cellular diagnostic test for uterine cancer. While conducting this research, he noticed that precancerous cells appeared in the exfoliation of vaginal fluid.[77]

He announced his initial findings related to cervical cancer in 1928 at the Third Race Betterment Conference. Papanicolaou explained that he could recognize malignant cells in a simple test: one could remove fluid from a woman's vagina, smear it on a slide, stain it, and study it. Precancerous cells became manifested in the exfoliation that appeared in the vaginal fluid.[78] His 1928 paper generated little response due to the strong conviction among cancer specialists that biopsy offered the only clear indication of cancer.[79] As one reviewer wrote, "Laboratory men were firm in their belief that the only dependable morphologic method for the diagnosis of cancer was that of the microscopic examination of a biopsy specimen and the evaluation of the architectural pattern of the cells in relation to each other."[80] As historian Eftychia Vayena has noted, "The response to this theory was indifferent or negative."[81]

Papanicolaou returned from this conference and engaged in a variety of studies in the 1930s. In late 1939, at the urging of the chair of the Cornell Department of Anatomy, Papanicolaou began collaborating with a specialist in gynecological pathology, Herbert Traut.[82] The two men studied the vaginal cells of women admitted to the hospital. Traut and Papanicolaou gained funding from the Commonwealth Fund and studied over 10,000 vaginal smears taken from more than 3,000 women.[83] By 1943, Traut and Papanicolaou had collected enough data to publish their influential work on cervical cancer and the diagnostic value of vaginal smears. *Diagnosis of Uterine Cancer by the Vaginal Smear* finally gained the attention of the medical and scientific community.[84] In 1948 Papanicolaou published "The Cell Smear Method of Diagnosing Cancer." Based on seven years of studies conducted at the Women's Clinic of New York Hospital, the study emphasized the importance of the smear technique, including the fixation of cells, precautions against drying out cells, and the adoption of his staining method. Papanicolaou anticipated the potential benefits of universal screening; however, he wrote, "This is a dream which cannot be realized at present."[85]

Several prominent physicians repeated these studies, ultimately confirming positive results of this screening technology.[86] Papanicolaou's research proved that cancerous and precancerous cells appeared in vaginal smears; theoretically, cervical cancer could be now prevented with medical intervention.[87] This research thus ushered in an era of preventive care through screening technology that revolutionized the mortality from cervical cancer in the United States.[88]

Papanicolaou's scientific discoveries coincided with major changes occurring within the American Cancer Society. ACS programming, such as the promotion of the breast self-examination film, reflected the organization's continued emphasis on early detection. In addition, beginning in 1946, the medical and scientific director of the ACS, Charles Cameron, wanted to demonstrate the ACS's new commitment to cancer research. Cameron befriended Papanicolaou and supported his research in the laboratory. Simultaneously, Cameron encouraged the development of early screening programs for uterine cancer within the female community.

With the support of the ACS and the confirmation of his results by other scientists, Papanicolaou's smear (commonly referred to as the

"Pap smear") became the most "successful" screening test for cancer to date.[89] As Dr. Papanicolaou explained in 1948, "The possibility of detecting early asymptomatic or hidden carcinomas by the smear technique has been convincingly proved, particularly for cervical carcinomas, by a rather impressive number of reports."[90] *Newsweek* elucidated the test to a wider audience: "Under careful microscopic examination, it is claimed, cancer cells in the vaginal secretion may be detected." By its conclusion, the *Newsweek* article expressed doubt over the effectiveness of this test, but it acknowledged the significant demand—"women patients have bombarded doctors with demands for the test."[91]

The first wave of enthusiasm for the Pap smear created unintended consequences. The more that journalists wrote about the vaginal smear in the mid-1940s, the more that public demand for the test soared. It soon became clear that the American medical community was unprepared for the mass screening of the female population. The U.S. health-care system lacked an infrastructure of equipped diagnostic centers, cancer specialists, and funds to support this effort. Moreover, few pathologists had training in cervical cytology. As demand continued to outpace supply, the ACS complained, "It was unfortunate indeed when some over-enthusiastic and unscientific members of the lay press announced the discovery in highly dramatic phraseology."[92] As the ACS and others realized, the implementation of any mass screening program would require huge sums of money to support medical training and the cost of medical services.

In 1948 the ACS sponsored a Cytological Diagnostic Conference that allowed for a discussion of this procedure and fostered a dialogue among groups of scientists about the value of smear technology. Part of the meeting focused on issues of public awareness and plans to meet the increased demand for the vaginal examination. By the end of the meeting, a resolution was passed that would discourage a publicity campaign, at least until more personnel could be trained in this procedure.

More than a decade passed before the ACS and cancer activists felt adequately prepared to launch a widespread promotion of the vaginal smear. This long delay suggests the different set of circumstances that surrounded cancer screening and prevention. Self-examinations, such as the BSE, did not require enormous funds or materials. Instead, women concerned about female health issues could create networks of information and learn about performing the BSE. The Pap smear, in contrast, required a formal infrastructure, financial support, and access to medical clinics and screening locations. The decade of transition between the idea of mass screening and its implementation exposed the limits of female volunteerism and women's increasing disfranchisement from important decisions about cancer control. Whereas the ACS encouraged the creation of the Women's Field Army that would control mass education programs throughout the 1930s and early 1940s, by midcentury female cancer educators lacked the financial and political clout necessary to shape cancer policy related to technology and screening.

The release of a popular cancer education film in 1957, *Time and Two Women*, marked the establishment of cervical cancer detection clinics, the training of pathologists in vaginal smears, and the wider application of this diagnostic procedure. The film indicated a level of preparedness within the ACS as it directed publicity to the exam and finally asked its female volunteers to promote it. By the late 1950s, demands for the diagnostic exams might be matched with equipped centers and trained staff.

Time and Two Women told the dramatic story of two women diagnosed with cervical cancer. Narrated by Dr. Joseph Meigs, an eminent gynecologist, this twenty-minute film offered a narrative description of uterine cancer.[93] Predictably, one story traces the experience of a fifty-two-year-old white woman who had had her last pelvic examination five years earlier. The postmenopausal woman insists, "I've never had any female trouble until now," and then recounts her recent episodes of vaginal bleeding, intense enough to last for five to six days and heavy enough to require up to twelve pads a day. The underlying theme of this storyline was the difficulty of curing cancer in its late stages.

Part of the film used animation to depict symptoms of cervical cancer. In the animation the uterus bleeds continually, and the viewer is forced to stare at the distracting and disturbing symptoms that this woman has chosen to ignore. At the conclusion of this mini-saga, Meigs holds up the patient's file. A large stamp on the front of it reads, "Deceased." Clearly, this film placed a sense of blame on women who ignored irregular vaginal discharge or unusual vaginal bleeding, the most obvious signs of uterine cancer. Like breast cancer, the best chance for treating reproductive cancer occurred in its early stage. Although women could not perform pelvic examinations on themselves, they could recognize irregular vaginal discharge or bleeding and seek prompt medical treatment.[94]

The film then details the story of another woman whose file lies on a larger stack of "cured" patient records. This middle-aged white woman visits her physician annually, even though she has no medical abnormalities. Rather, she has complied with suggestions for regular pelvic examinations. The film delineates the steps involved in a vaginal smear. Several scenes are devoted to explaining that this woman's routine vaginal smear has revealed the very early stages of uterine cancer. She learns that, just like the woman who has died, her "cancer" had started in the cervix. The second woman's diagnosis was not devastating, however, because the vaginal smear has revealed precancerous cells. Conflating the distinction between precancerous cells and cancer, the film implicitly created parallels between different types of cancer detection.[95] The message to viewers is obvious: she survived because Dr. Meigs discovered these cells in their earliest stages. The film celebrates the compliant patient and the authoritative physician.

This film reflected postwar trends in cancer education that assumed that medical expertise could now "cure" cancer. Moreover, it maintained an implicit assumption that women who delayed visits to the doctor could be blamed for their late-stage diagnosis. More widespread use of the word "cure," however imprecise, stemmed from the emerging rhetoric of solution and effective treatment. Popular discourse generally ignored scientific controversy regarding the likelihood of recurrence and burgeoning disputes about the effectiveness of cancer treatment, the need for radical operations, and the disempowerment of patients in cancer decisions.[96]

Clearly, Papanicolaou's studies that revealed that precancerous cells could be discovered without surgery relieved many apprehensions about diagnostic procedures for uterine cancer. Ultimately, cancer awareness advocates would advise women to schedule annual physical examinations that included both a vaginal smear and a breast examination. Not surprisingly, much of the rhetoric about the late diagnosis of uterine cancer soon sounded like that of breast cancer, depicting women who died as victims of their modesty.

Race/Ethnicity and Cancer: Efforts to Recognize Patterns

By midcentury, growing concern for reproductive cancers coincided with federal efforts to track cancer mortality. Between 1950 and 1952 the U.S. Public Heath Service published reports that compared cancer morbidity in ten major cities. This study compared cancer data among different population groups, specifically comparing cancer in African American and white populations. Although statistics showed that cancer occurred more frequently in white populations, a comparison by anatomical sites demonstrated that black women had higher rates of breast and cervical cancer than white women.[97] The *Cancer Morbidity Series* also stressed the notable difference in morbidity from reproductive cancers among African American women.[98]

For centuries minority health issues had been marginalized in the dominant discourse about health care in the United States. At best, the health concerns confronting communities of color were ignored. At worst, medical professionals violated communities of color and cultivated a culture of distrust and suspicion of medical services.[99] The issue of race in American medicine pervaded discussions of cancer in the early twentieth century. As Frederick Hoffman, the most prominent statistician for cancer in the early 1900s, noted, "The element of race in cancer mortality has previously been referred to as a matter of exceptional interest and importance." Although his data varied by the type of cancer and age, he argued that "white death-rates are considerably in excess."[100]

Physicians who were concerned with African American health care stressed the misleading nature of these assertions as early as the 1920s. Dr. Louis Wright, one of the first black graduates of Harvard University Medical School and founder of the Cancer Research Center at Harlem Hospital, argued that Hoffman's data ignored disparities in record keeping among different racial groups in the United States. It failed to consider the early average age of death among the black population and ignored the likelihood of improper diagnoses. Wright urged statisticians to compare cancer by site and to factor in the impact of race on cancer statistics.[101] As early as 1937, in a statistical study of cancer among the African American population, James Moseley aptly noted, "It should be apparent that the attack on such a problem as this cannot end with the mere dissemination of knowledge about cancer, but must aim to furnish more adequate medical care as a preventive against the results of neglect."[102]

But with a few notable exceptions, in the late 1940s cancer awareness efforts continued to concentrate on mass dissemination of cancer information. Moreover, the narratives and images portrayed in these publications reflected the dominant American culture of a white and middle-class population.[103] Cancer awareness programs targeted privileged white, educated, and middle-class women. Although educational efforts varied and included more widespread use of educational films, the reliance on early detection as a preventive model proved consistent and compelling. Cancer activists, especially members of the ACS, insisted that informing women of the importance of early detection could save countless lives. As *Ladies' Home Journal* proclaimed, "WOMEN NEED NO LONGER DIE of Their No. 1 Cancer Foe!"[104] Statements such as this were framed by assumptions about women's access to health care and women's faith in medical services. Disproportionately, women of color could not afford health services, and many did not trust medical professionals. Midcentury formal cancer education programs failed to respond to these circumstances.

The release of the U.S. Public Health Service survey in 1952 responded to some of Mosely's and Wright's concerns and directed some overdue attention to African American health, particularly to the high rate of reproductive cancers among African American women. By midcentury, more medical studies were documenting the disparity in cancer morbidity by race. Although popular educational literature did little to publicize these trends, some scientific teams argued that the government needed to explore the connections between socioeconomic status and cancer more carefully. As one team concluded, "The remarkably higher relative frequency of cervical cancer in the Negro previously reported is not the result of racial susceptibility but rather is associated with factors relative to the lower socioeconomic status of the Negro in the United States."[105] Most cancer educators, however, continued to merely reassert the value and importance of early detection.

With the notable exception of the National Council of Negro Women, there was limited response to the alarmingly high rates of cervical cancer among African American women. In fact, the regular monthly publication of the American Cancer Society, *Cancer News*, which recorded many local achievements in cancer awareness for both breast and reproductive cancers, included no reports of programs that targeted African Americans. Likewise, education efforts failed to target Hispanic or Asian women. Moreover, popular cancer literature continued to use images of white women. As a result, African American women organized themselves and discussed the risk of cancer, but they frequently had little choice but to rely on educational materials that featured white women.

Despite the race-specific nature of much of the ACS teaching material, some African American women created their own space within the organization. In 1939 Alice B. Crutcher organized a "Colored Division" within the Women's Field Army. Working through the Federation of Colored Women's Clubs, she established twenty-eight units throughout Kentucky that targeted the African American community. As the 1942–43 Kentucky Division annual report read, "No group of workers has been more enthusiastic, faithful, willing, and conscientious than the Colored Unit, and we congratulate these women on their excellent achievement." Similarly, in 1950, when the ACS launched the breast self-examination project, the Oregon State Federation of Colored Women's Clubs cooperated. The federation hosted film viewings, invited African American doctors to serve on its speakers' bureau, and organized meetings for black women seeking information on cancer. As these programs suggest, African American women worked with the resources available to teach black communities about cancer.[106]

Comparing Models of Care

It is telling to compare and contrast the shifts in screening programs for uterine/cervical and breast cancer. Both stressed early detection, placed the burden of early detection on women, and implied that women who delayed detection played a role in their eventual death from the disease. These similarities notwithstanding, the diagnostic procedure for each was quite different. Women could perform breast self-examination at home, but a vaginal smear could only be done by a medical professional in an office, clinic, or hospital. The breast self-examination was free; vaginal smears were costly.

Despite these obvious differences, the press, especially women's magazines, persisted in emphasizing the parallels of these different cancer detection methods for the popular audiences. Noticeably, by 1960, the rhetoric of performing a breast self-examination monthly and getting a Pap smear annually portrayed the woman as executing important diagnostic steps. Clearly, however, a woman played a much more active role in a BSE than in a vaginal smear. In addition, popular literature blurred the scientific disparity between these two dissimilar diagnostic procedures and maintained the rhetoric that women needed to detect their cancer if treatment were to be effective. Significantly, the popular literature did not expose the uncertainties of screening technology and criticism of false results in testing. Instead, by painting women as pivotal actors in the diagnosis of both breast and cervical cancer in the postwar years, educators created the illusion that individual women were empowered to combat cancer.

Early detection offered promise for decreasing cancer fatalities, but it did not offer the cure that much of the literature suggested. In 1945 the Gallup Poll reported that 62 percent of people surveyed believed cancer was curable if caught in time. In 1950, 60 percent of people surveyed believed cancer was curable. Three years later, 65 percent responded that they believed cancer was curable. The poll data suggests that cancer educators may well have given the public a false optimism.[107]

Much of this information was buttressed by the visual images that film offered. Lisa Cartwright argues in *Screening the Body* that "scientific knowledge and scientific subjectivities are resolutely entangled with a broad range and mix of cultural and representational practices." She emphasizes that film cannot be interpreted within a single context but must include multiple analyses of the social and cultural influences that shape the viewer.[108] Women who watched the *Breast Self-Examination* usually did so in an all-female audience, in the company of a "medical expert," who stressed the power and innovation of this examination. Although some watched the film in large urban movie houses, and others collected in small local women's clubs, all viewers felt the camaraderie of women who shared similar medical concerns. One can speculate that they easily envisioned the exam as the potent new weapon it was labeled in this era of technological innovation. Film offered a visual image filled with instruction, but more important, it fostered a firmer sense of community among women who were aware of the risk breast cancer posed in midlife.

In addition, the shift to autobiographical stories in this period, used mainly in popular magazine articles but also evident in films such as *Choose to Live*, dramatized individual reactions to cancer and diagnosis. Patterns evident in these autobiographies suggested common concerns for women (mastectomy, metastasis, death) and shared strategies for coping with the disease (consulting experts, disguising the mastectomy). Surely, it lessened the sense of isolation some women may have experienced when diagnosed. Unlike the powerful personal rhetoric of the women's health movement in the 1970s, however, these autobiographical and individual narratives did not translate into political activism in the 1950s.

Conclusion

Historians need to cast a more critical eye on this concept of false modesty among women and cancer in the twentieth century. It is obvious that by midcentury large numbers of women had learned about cancer, discussed it among themselves, and organized to teach it to a broader audience. They watched films about the breast self-examination in urban theaters surrounded by hundreds of other viewers. Certainly, some women felt discomfort with the medical profession and issues of reproductive health. As one woman explained, "I don't care to see any gynecologist. I loathe having them prodding and poking at me. All I'm having are a few simple signs of menopause."[109] Yet these anecdotal references suggest an anxiety about the profession and patient-physician interaction. Such reactions fostered the sense that patients simply needed to learn more about early detection (to overcome their reluctance to see their doctor) and ignored emerging debates within the medical professional about treatment, the emphasis on self-examinations and increased anxiety about cancer, and the limitations of screening technology.

Cancer has long been defined as a disease without discrimination, affecting people of any class, gender, or race. Yet an overview of the breast and cervical awareness campaigns in the late 1940s and early 1950s demonstrates how these categories defined cancer, the women who were targeted by the education campaigns, and the programs designed to decrease the incidence of cancer. The breast cancer awareness programs approached privileged white, middle- and upper-class women, often women involved in club work, philanthropy, and reform. Although the ACS articulated a concern for educating minority women, its reports on the success of raising breast cancer awareness chronicled its success in reaching a white audience.[110] In the late 1940s and early 1950s, female educators articulated concerns about cancers peculiar to their sex, but many failed to recognize how the categories of race, class, and gender shaped their education and research agendas. Clearly, these education programs, which were meant to teach all women about breast cancer and reproductive cancers, lacked cultural specificity and ignored the unequal access to health care in a system based on privatized medicine.

Finally, the focus on early detection may have hindered a sophisticated discussion of treatment and the long-term effects of cancer treatment. The three distinct narrative patterns of the postwar years—stories that featured two women with opposite reactions to their initial cancer symptoms; lessons of effective early detection visually depicted in educational films; and a shift to more autobiographical stories—continued to focus almost exclusively on early detection. Narratives conveyed the story of opposites by highlighting the "wisdom" of women who detected cancer early and survived the disease versus the naiveté of women who ignored cancer symptoms and subsequently died of the disease. One author explained, "Breast cancer is a killer primarily because women put off the visit to their doctor for weeks and even years—they dread the diagnosis, dread mysterious treatment, dread disfigurement."[111] Without known cures for cancer, this rhetoric informed women of a temporary solution: assume responsibility for your health, overcome modesty about your body, and follow doctor's advice about prevention and treatment for female cancers.

4

Cancer Survivors

PUBLIC DISCUSSIONS OF
POSTDIAGNOSTIC CONCERNS

Throughout the twentieth century, public messages about cancer stressed the value of early detection. In the postwar era, however, cancer narratives, especially those directed to female audiences, also began to address postdiagnostic concerns. Specifically, cancer education films, popular women's magazine articles, and women's club meetings increasingly recognized a population of cancer survivors and their shared concerns. Moving beyond the early diagnosis stage, these illness narratives described women's sense of loss after a mastectomy, a fear of recurrence after treatment, and personal reactions to cancer treatment. In the second half of the century, a more nuanced and complicated version of female cancers appeared in popular education material that explored experiences after cancer treatment.

For decades white women had learned about their risk of breast cancer and the importance of early detection. Until midcentury, however, public discussion of the consequences of mastectomy and the challenges of survival remained a mystery for much of the lay public. Beginning in the mid-1950s cancer awareness material became more intimate, including information about the effects of treatment, reactions to cancer surgery, and anxiety shared by many patients who feared metastasis. Women diagnosed with breast cancer in particular began to talk about the sense of loss that accompanied a mastectomy, and narrative patterns emerged in these women's stories that reflected shared concerns about the body, emotions, and treatment. These shared concerns would foster a collective consciousness among women who critiqued standard medical treatment.

This chapter examines the emerging sense of community forged among cancer survivors in midcentury. As historian Anne Firor Scott has demonstrated, uncovering local women's activism and community movements offers a lens through which to better understand social frameworks of the past.[1] The community of women who joined the ACS demonstrated commitment to its educational mission, especially its goal of teaching women about cancer risks. For some, this meant screenings of the *Breast Self-Examination* film during lunchtime in western mill towns, while for others it meant entering classrooms to tell children about the disease. As illustrated by a brief case study of cancer education in Cedar Rapids, Iowa, the effort played out differently in urban and rural environments. In Cedar Rapids and elsewhere, male physicians played critical roles in cancer education campaigns; yet, physicians depended on women to educate the public. Moreover, this case study exposes the cooperative impulses among female lay educators and male physicians who both embraced early detection as the best means to controlling this devastating illness.

The American Cancer Society and Early Detection Scenarios

In 1946 the American Cancer Society (ACS) produced the film *Time Is Life*. Like earlier films produced by the ACS, it stressed the value of early detection for women, insisted that women needed to respond to any early indications of cancer, and suggested that the public did not talk about cancer enough. But unlike prior films, *Time Is Life* offered audiences a detailed discussion of the medical procedures that accompanied a breast cancer diagnosis. Expanding the medical discussion of breast cancer treatment for lay audiences, this film identified postsurgical concerns. Likewise, it recognized that a community of women had experienced and survived the procedure.[2]

Time Is Life opens with ominous music and the somber tone of a narrator who explains that Mary Bronson, "a worried housewife," discovered "what might be" a symptom of cancer one week ago. Mary is unable to sleep and worries about what will happen if she has cancer. "Will I die?" she wonders. As she ambles around her home in the middle of the night, she explains, "People don't tell you about cancer. They don't talk about it. Why not? Is there no hope . . . no hope?" Throughout the film these thoughts of cancer distract Bronson from her daily routine. The film emphasizes Bronson's confusion, fear, and sense of isolation.

Bronson eventually enters a local ACS office, where a female member of the Field Army explains early symptoms of cancer.[3] The ACS volunteer encourages Bronson to seek medical attention since this response may save her life. After most of this drama has played out, the viewer finally learns that Bronson's concern stems from a lump in her breast.

The role played by the female volunteer in this film does more than facilitate a narrative. It normalizes the intimacy that women shared when discussing matters of their health and bodies. In fact, Bronson's opportunity to visit an ACS office stemmed from the decades since 1913 when women devised ways to reach a broader audience and promulgate the message of early detection.[4] In virtually every ACS film created for female audiences, female volunteers served as mediators between the medical profession and the patient.

Time Is Life shifts from an emotional story to a medical one as Bronson learns that "cancer is often curable if treated in time." Typical of popular cancer awareness material, the film lists the seven major warning signs of cancer. A male doctor explains to the viewer why Bronson needs a medical examination, the role of "science fighting by her side," the rapid growth of cancer cells, and the danger they pose to the human body. He compares the behavior of cancer to that of a "gangster." Such aggressive imagery emphasizes the dangers of untreated cancer, while the voice of the authoritative doctor claiming the power of science for the patient insists that physicians can treat cancer.

The physician then explains the biopsy procedure, surgical treatment, and the purpose of adjuvant x-ray and radium treatment. The doctor encourages Bronson to permit a complete mastectomy if the cancer is present. At this point, Bronson (and the viewer) have images of cancer's growth in their mind; music with quick tempo reminds the viewer that action must be prompt and insinuates that patients who delay are needlessly making themselves vulnerable. Within this context Bronson "readily" agrees to a complete mastectomy if necessary.[5]

The film dramatizes the time that elapses between the biopsy and Bronson's mastectomy. A ticking clock is featured while the surgeon awaits the pathology report—clearly symbolizing the importance of wasting no time if one suspects cancer. The narrator articulates the obvious concern: "Will a vitally important cancer operation be performed?" Mary Bronson is under anesthesia throughout, and the film shows how a tissue sample is frozen, sliced, dyed, and studied. A brief discussion of treatment options, if the tissue is malignant, follows. Even as this film introduced the public to a broader discussion of cancer treatment, it continued to accentuate the importance of time and implicitly applauded a one-step and radical mastectomy procedure.[6]

Time Is Life then shifts its focus to the laboratory where the pathologist deems Bronson's tissue healthy, and her "ugly, nagging fear" can be put to rest. More important, the viewer has learned the procedural steps involved in a diagnosis. Finally, the narrator has informed the viewer that surgery, radium, and x-ray can treat a cancer discovered in its early stage.

This near-cancer experience inspires Bronson to engage in cancer awareness, and she encourages a neighbor to seek medical advice if she is concerned about cancer. The messages of the film are threefold. First, do not worry about cancer but face it, and visit a doctor at the first symptom of the disease. Second, do not feel ashamed and isolated when confronting cancer. Anyone and everyone is susceptible to it. Finally, learn about the medical procedures for cancer and appreciate that treatment can be effective, especially if the cancer is discovered early. Although the primary purpose of the film was educational, it also likely served to recruit more female volunteers. The foot soldier image introduced in the 1930s with the Women's Field Army resonated for years to come as women volunteered their time and energy to talk with one another about a dreaded disease.

The film also nodded at women's conversations with each other about cancer experiences. Closing scenes show Bronson talking with a neighbor about cancer. It is impossible to historically recreate the numerous conversations that women shared with neighbors, family, and friends after a biopsy or diagnosis. Anecdotal evidence suggests that women had conversations about their fears but that the majority trusted the medical doctrine of early detection. Many of these women opted to work within organized groups such as the ACS to promote it.

Public Discussion of Treatment

In early 1951 *Ladies' Home Journal* published "Diagnosis: Cancer, Recovery, Probable." Similar to the 1946 ACS film, this article explored cancer treatment and the anxiety that surrounded it. The author, Lily MacLeod, had recently been diagnosed with advanced cervical cancer. She described her experience in detail, which included the paternalistic attitude of her doctor, discomfort and pain from radiation treatment, and the anguish of learning that treatment had been ineffective. She also recognized the chance for recurrence. In a departure from many cancer narratives, MacLeod offered a glimpse of the aftermath of her cancer diagnosis. She openly shared her sense of unease after surgery, caused by a looming and constant possibility of recurrence and death. Moving beyond single messages of early detection, postwar literature now recognized the experiences of cancer survivors.

MacLeod began the story with her initial experiences of abnormal vaginal bleeding that had inspired her to visit to a gynecologist. "The examination which followed was startlingly painful. When the doctor touched a certain spot it felt as though he had used a branding iron. I stiffened and cried out," she wrote. She soon learned that she had an ulcer at the mouth of her womb, her entire cervix was raw and inflamed, and the doctor had removed some tissue for a biopsy. Meanwhile, the doctor "left the end of the table and came to my side, drawing the sheet away from my breasts. I felt his fingers probing and he gave me a little smile. 'You're safe *there*, anyhow.'" This offhand remark accentuated the distance between physicians and patients, but it also encouraged audiences to make parallels between breast and cervical cancer.[7]

MacLeod did in fact have cancer and started x-ray treatment immediately. As she explained, "I lost possession of my body. It became the property of my doctors—and my cancer." X-ray treatment for cervical cancer entailed external treatment, internal treatment, or a combination of both. Making a choice in her medical treatment, MacLeod opted for the most promising treatment (as described by the physician), combination therapy. As medical treatment options expanded in the second half of the twentieth century, patients gained some agency in determining their treatment.[8]

Internal treatment consisted of the doctor's inserting a cone-shaped device into the vagina. MacLeod apparently expressed apprehension about the procedure, as the doctor commented, "Don't look so scared. It won't be painful. Unpleasant at first, for it must go in and be carefully adjusted." MacLeod's experience validated his description. As she wrote, "there was a certain amount of manipulation necessary to adjust it, but except for the actual placement there was no real discomfort." During external treatment, a radiologist directed radiation toward MacLeod's pelvis. On alternate days the rays would be aimed through the waist or the back. MacLeod explained the minute details of her x-ray treatment, describing both the physical characteristics of the radiation machine and the medical practitioners involved.[9]

MacLeod also wrote about her emotional reaction to the cervical cancer diagnosis. She described her fears and regrets, identified her new sense of self, questioned her relationship to technology, and wondered about her participation in medical treatment. She dreaded explaining her diagnosis and treatment to her mother and daughter. MacLeod's narrative thus embodied the midcentury shift in popular cancer literature beyond morality tales of delaying diagnosis and toward a more nuanced discussion of individual experiences with a cancer diagnosis and personal reactions to cancer treatment.

After her first round of treatment, MacLeod returned for a medical checkup. "The instant he touched my cervix I had a sense of foreboding," she related. "It was very painful. Almost as painful as the first examination in his office had been." MacLeod learned that the cancer was still present and that one treatment alternative existed—radium. Complicating the scenario of early detection and assured cure, this narrative began with early detection, described failed treatment, and recognized alternative treatment options.

The alternative treatment option involved a process whereby a physician would insert capsules of radium into MacLeod's vagina. The capsules would remain in place for several days, hopefully destroying the cancer cells. MacLeod described the great bouts of pain that she experienced as a result of this treatment. She felt burning sensations in her back and aches in her body. She later learned that "Dr. T" had used a new procedure on her that might have provoked the pain, undermining any sense of agency that MacLeod may have gained in choosing her treatment and agreeing to an alternative therapy. After some time, MacLeod finally felt well, and her health seemed restored.

Although MacLeod's story has a happy ending, the significance of her narrative can be found in her description of physician-patient relations. MacLeod believed that doctors should tell women all the details of their diagnosis and treatment. "Much of my own mental agony was the unknown," she wrote. "In telling my story I tried, to the best of my ability, to draw a picture of a woman who has fought cancer and lived to tell the tale."[10] MacLeod's narrative highlights the trend toward a public discussion of comprehensive stories of cancer diagnoses and treatment, stories that included details of pain and reactions to unsuccessful treatment. It also alludes to emerging criticism of the medical profession and to a patient's early assertion of her right to decide about treatment.

Edna Kaehele published a similar article in *Woman's Home Companion* a year later, "I Am Living with Cancer," describing her struggle to survive stomach cancer. This author did not claim that she was cured; instead, she embraced the idea that her cancer experience was embedded in her sense of identity. Kaehele's experience with surgery and radiation transformed her life and her relationship with technology, which she described as "the fantastic machinery that was to become so familiar in the next few months."[11]

As a final example of the emerging trends in cancer narratives, in 1953 a reader asked, "Did you ever hear of a woman seventy-one years old starting to menstruate again?" In "Tell Me Doctor," a feature column of *Ladies' Home Journal*, the columnist responded that irregular vaginal bleeding could indicate several problems and that the reader needed to seek medical consultation. The columnist then described one procedure that could reveal the source of the blood, "a diagnostic curettage, a thorough scraping of the uterine interior which I hope will provide the answer to our problem." Whereas earlier cancer articles had often alluded to vague medical procedures, postwar articles often described the process for lay audiences. To be sure, articles continued to insist that early detection often made the difference between life and death. In addition to describing the procedure, this columnist wrote, "Cancer does not always wear a big *C* sign on its breast. When we come down to the final denominator, cancer is cancer, and a wholesome respect for it is wise. The penalty for any error is tragic."[12] Yet by midcentury, popular cancer narratives included a more comprehensive description of the medical procedures and began to recognize the difficulties of curing the disease.

By the middle of the decade, detailed discussions of treatment became increasingly common. *Woman's Home Companion* published "If the Verdict Is Cancer" in 1955. The subtitle read, "What will happen to you if your doctor finds you have cancer? Here for the first time a cancer expert leads you through this dreaded experience step by step." The step-by-step instruction appeared in similar women's magazine throughout the mid-1950s. The author's byline, which listed his affiliation with the Department of Preventative Medicine of the Memorial Center for Cancer and Allied Diseases, the Strang Cancer Prevention Clinic, and the New York City Cancer Committee, suggested that medical professionals willingly participated in this effort to expand the popular discussion of cancer treatment. As author Emerson Day noted of one female patient, "She had been warned to catch signs of cancer early but she had never been told what would happen to her if cancer were discovered."[13]

Day spelled out what a woman might experience after she discovered a suspicious lump in her breast. A biopsy procedure usually included at least one night in the hospital, general anesthesia, and the minor pain associated with a needle prick that rendered the patient unconscious for the procedure. He then explained the one-step procedure, whereby a biopsy specimen was sent immediately to pathology. If the sample was deemed benign, the woman returned to her room to recover. If, however, it was cancerous, a radical mastectomy was performed on the spot: "Working slowly and carefully, the team of surgeons first separate the breast tissues from the muscles of the chest wall. Although all of the inside of the breast is removed, a portion of its surface skin is retained to help cover the area. Then they remove the two muscles in the hollow of your shoulder and the lymph glands of the armpit which have been found to be a common path for cancer cells to follow in spreading from the breasts to other parts of the body."[14] Day also described the expected size, shade, and shape of the scar and offered details about when it might heal. He dealt briefly with the psychological aspects of mastectomy but tended to rely on stereotypical and gendered notions about women and their reaction to losing a breast: "Reactions are never the same in each patient—all of us are individuals. But most women, to a greater or lesser degree, develop the fear that their femininity has been endangered. If you are married you may worry that your husband will not accept your 'mutilated' state. If you are single you may envision yourself no longer able to compete with other women for a husband."[15]

Finally, Day described radiation as painless. A woman would remove her clothes and lie on a cot, and an operator stationed outside the room would turn on the radiation machine. Days after the treatment, the author warned, a woman might sense a slight skin burn, queasiness, or mild diarrhea. He also included a quick summary of hormonal treatment, a less popular treatment for breast cancer but one that was gaining some followers in the 1950s. Although this physician assumed a factual tone, his candor about surgery reflected postwar trends to inform patients about cancer treatment. However, his descriptions may have distorted the reality of cancer treatment and its harmful effects on the body. For example, he described radiation as "painless," obscuring the postsurgical discomfort associated with the treatment.

"These 7 People Were Saved From Cancer," published in *Ladies' Home Journal* in March 1957, celebrated cancer survivors, including one woman who was treated successfully for breast cancer and another for cervical cancer. The woman with breast cancer had surgery: "Her right breast was removed, and the surrounding tissue all the way to the lymph glands under the right arm. Cancer surgery must often be radical. The rapidly growing, disordered cells invade everywhere. To hope for a cure, the surgeons must remove every last cell." The woman with cervical cancer experienced x-ray treatment and then a seven-hour surgery to remove her uterus.[16] Like Day's article, this piece reflected the dominant medical model that advocated extensive surgery and informed the reader of the extent of the excision and the duration of the surgery. Embedded within these discussions of cancer treatment was the pervasive image of hope and optimism.

A little over a year later, in May 1958, the front cover of *Life* magazine featured a woman lying on her back, covered in white hospital sheets, staring upward toward a large radiation machine that was several times her size and occupied 80 percent of the cover. A caption to the left of the supine woman read, "2,000,000 volt radiation for cancer patient." The accompanying article promised, "Fresh Hope on Cancer: 12 Pages on the Newest Methods to Save You from Malignancies." Although this article sensationalized new forms of energy as potential anticancer agents, it also highlighted the real problem of cancer malignancy. Surgical treatments alone seemed unable to yield the promised cure, but the story suggested that new forms of energy might.[17]

"No matter how perfect methods become," the text read, they are pointless unless successful treatment can follow." Much of the article praised advances in radiation that could be administered "from gigantic x-ray machines, atom smashers, atomic isotopes and even nuclear reactors."[18] This and other stories clearly employed the rhetoric of nuclear science and exaggerated the value of radiation therapy. Frequent references to the technology's size and attributes seemed to suggest an improved form of cancer control, but they also revealed the rise of alternative treatments and alluded to some dissension within the medical profession. Although these stories overstated the machine's potential, they contributed to the expanding public discussion of nonsurgical treatment options.

After Treatment: Prosthesis and Reach to Recovery

Marion Flexner's autobiographical story, "Cancer—I've Had It," published in 1947, offered one of the first popular discussions of breast prosthesis. Flexner shared her opinions about this artificial part: "One of my first problems was to get a false breast, which I knew I would have to wear as soon as I put my clothes on. I called a local department store and ordered one over the telephone. It came—a small, pincushionlike affair to be shoved into the empty side of my old brassiere."[19] The "falsie," however, did not fit. Moreover, it failed to resemble a human breast. She then visited a "surgical *corsetiere*" and bought a false breast made of sponge rubber. This form served its purpose; it resembled a breast and restored Flexner's confidence. The emerging market for prosthetic breasts suggests that Flexner's postsurgical concerns about the acquisition of a prosthesis were shared by other breast cancer survivors. As American culture captured a broader discussion of treatment options and concerns about surgery, it also began exploring women's reactions to losing a breast.

There is a long history of breast prosthesis production in the United States. As early as 1874 the government issued the first patent for a breast form, and since then over 228 patents categorized as an artificial breast have been filed.[20] These patents reflect the variety of concerns associated with this artificial part, including its weight, comfort, appearance, and durability. As early as 1906, one designer recommended a casing made of rubber because it could "be colored and otherwise treated to lend the same realistic appearance." In 1922 another inventor described the importance of "a convenient and comfortable substitute for the bust of a woman, which has been removed by surgical operation." At least somewhat familiar with breast cancer survivors, this inventor suggested that the breast form consist of a silk casing, cushion fill, and a whale bone ring to maintain the shape of the artificial breast.[21] By 1937, several patents referred to the extensive "removal of breasts, muscle and flesh of the human body in the vicinity of the chest" associated with the radical mastectomy.[22] World War II and the scientific advances that it funded led to the discovery of synthetic chemicals that could alter the properties of products such as rubber. Ultimately, this contributed to the creation of a more practical breast substitute and transformed the breast prosthesis industry into a manufacturing business that catered to a specific audience of breast cancer survivors.

The story of the breast prosthesis tells more than a history of manufacture and business, however. It reflects the broadening popular discussions of cancer in American culture and a public dialogue about cancer survivors. Journalists and others assumed survivors would want to mask the results of their mastectomy. As midcentury journalist Maxine Davis noted, "No one outside the immediate family need know she has had the operation—just as she does not know that many women whose names are household words have undergone the experience."[23] Ironically, at the same time that cancer activists urged a more nuanced and open discussion of cancer and its treatments, literature about prostheses taught women how to hide the effects of their surgery. Although some women may have accepted such culturally sanctioned advice uncritically, others began to consider the ways that medicine and cancer awareness had failed women.

Throughout the 1950s, while American popular culture celebrated large breasts, writers examining cancer assumed that women needed prosthetic breasts after mastectomy. As Marilyn Yalom has written, "What meanings we give our breasts will always be bound up with societal values and cultural norms."[24] Maxine Davis dispensed typical advice: "As soon as the doctor gives his permission, the patient should be fitted with a prosthetic device called a breast form, available in most good department stores and specialty shops. If possible she should consult a good *corsetiere* who has had experience with this problem. Many stores employ women who themselves have had mastectomy, to help customers." Such discussions of prosthetic breasts reflected the growing product line available by midcentury. "The device may be made of plain rubber, foam rubber, liquid-filled plastic, or air-filled plastic. It should match the remaining breast as closely as possible, at the sides, front, and top."[25] Manufacturers tapped into the sizable population of breast cancer patients and anticipated profits by selling to this discrete community.

In addition to providing information about the material culture of the breast prosthesis and advice about purchasing it, postwar popular literature began discussing the psychological impact of losing a breast. Many experts concluded that the prosthetic form had healing powers that could eventually restore women's sense of balance and normalcy. As one woman shared, "The hardest lesson for me was how to cope with fear. For months *after* the mastectomy I lived in a new kind of terror. I had lost part of myself for which there could be no compensation—an integral part of my femininity. I hid away in my room, feeling like a criminal every time I put on my new foam-rubber breast. It seemed a sort of deception I was perpetuating on the general public because it allowed me to pretend to be a whole woman." Her narrative exposed the blurring of boundaries between medicine, culture, and identity. Concerns about postoperative care, ranging from restoring motion in the arm to assuring women that they could still be beautiful, captured important elements of patients' experiences. This woman articulated a sense of embarrassment that resulted from her mastectomy. "I would have preferred losing an arm or leg—something that could be discussed publicly without flinching—anything unconnected with sex," she admitted. Eventually, she claimed to gain a sense of "normalcy" by wearing the prosthesis, but she had opened a conversation with the reader about life after cancer treatment and the web of issues she confronted as a result.[26]

In "I'm Glad I Had My Breast Removed," the author revealed her reticence to discuss postmastectomy concerns with her male doctor. Her doctor finally introduced the subject and encouraged the author to wear a proper prosthesis after surgery. He explained, "Wearing an artificial breast . . . will give you the confidence and the pleasure of knowing you look perfectly natural to others." Reinforcing dominant cultural norms that identified a woman's sense of confidence with her breast image, the doctor's opinion resonated with the patient. She expressed relief when she described her first prosthesis fitting. "A nurse came and took my measurements," she wrote, "and by the time I was ready to leave the hospital my new brassieres were ready and waiting for me. The form was exactly like my other breast in size and shape, built to replace even the underarm fullness that was taken away. Its soft, pliable composition makes it feel natural against my body."[27]

Popular journals that addressed the issue of losing a breast universally urged women to disguise the mastectomy's results. The implications of this message, evident in most discussions of cancer treatment and recovery in the second half of the twentieth century, are steeped in the cultural norms of the 1950s, which valued women's full figures and a fashion style that emphasized large breasts. Cancer awareness advocates seemed committed to assuring women that life after cancer could be "normal," and normalcy seemed most tangible in its physical representations. Three decades later, Audre Lorde would remind audiences that prostheses served to disguise the impact of breast cancer and masked a visible reminder of its ubiquity in the United States.[28] But midcentury discussions in popular cancer awareness material did not recognize this possible critique and instead adjusted to dialogue that recognized the effects of mastectomy, discussed prosthesis experiences, and offered individual solutions to the community of breast cancer survivors.

From a medical and surgical perspective, most women who survived breast cancer lost one or both breasts in their entirety. Many women also lost part of their chest wall and surrounding tissue due to the extensive nature of radical mastectomy.[29] As women wrote about their reaction to the radical mastectomy and their breast amputations, many lamented the physical loss, especially in a culture that valorized women's breasts. In "I Had Breast Cancer," Terese Lasser referred to mastectomy when she wrote, "A deplorable curtain of silence hangs about this subject and it is time we lift it. . . . The taboos, the stigma, the absurd old wives' tales need to be exposed, and exploded."[30] She would begin to confront these issues by recognizing a community of breast cancer survivors with a group she formed in midcentury, Reach to Recovery.

Reach to Recovery

In March 1938 at the International Building of the Rockefeller Center in New York City, Dr. Anna C. Palmer announced the formation of a "Cured Cancer Club." Then eighty-one years old, Palmer had been a breast cancer survivor since 1920. As part of the opening celebration, Palmer urged cancer survivors to "come forward and show the world that cancer can be cured." Sharing the platform with influential leaders in the cancer movement, like American Society for the Control of Cancer (ASCC) director C. C. Little and Women's Field Army (WFA) national commander Marjorie Illig, Palmer served as president of this small club, which invited survivors of any type of cancer. Physicians had long discussed cancer survivors as a statistic, but with Palmer's announcement the public learned about a self-identified community of people who had survived cancer. Five other members of the club stood with Palmer at the Rockefeller Center, including cervical, larynx, lip, and breast cancer survivors.[31]

Almost two decades after the creation of the Cured Cancer Club, a larger and exclusively female cancer survivor community was formed.[32] Based on a similar concept to the Cured Cancer Club—the recognition of cancer survivors—Reach to Recovery, established in 1954, specifically offered support to women with breast cancer. Seeking to alleviate the isolation and individual dread that many women experienced upon diagnosis, founder Terese Lasser employed the language of shared experience to forge a communal identity for breast cancer survivors. Although the program was designed to facilitate one-on-one conversations for women diagnosed with breast cancer, its membership and publications emphasized that many women survived breast cancer. Moreover, breast cancer survivors were often willing to share their experiences with others.

Lasser envisioned Reach to Recovery as an organization that would help make intimate discussions of breast cancer and mastectomy possible. Reach to Recovery volunteers, limited to women who had experienced breast cancer themselves, first visited newly diagnosed women in the hospital. (During the one-step era, diagnosis and mastectomy usually occurred on the same day.) The volunteers would discuss the effects of mastectomy with patients, tell them about various breast prosthesis options, and teach exercises that restored arm mobility after such a radical surgery. Eventually, volunteers would offer to recently diagnosed women temporary artificial breasts as well. Based on the principle that women with similar diagnoses and treatment could best offer counsel, the Reach to Recovery program matched individual women who had survived breast cancer with women who were recovering from their mastectomy.

Lasser created this support network with fervor and dedication. She personally typed the first edition of the *Reach to Recovery: A Manual for Women Who Have Had Radical Breast Surgery* in 1953, bound it in a bright yellow cover, and distributed 10,000 copies. As Lasser explained in the foreword, "This manual has been prepared for the sole purpose of assisting you to achieve your maximum recovery—

physically, mentally, and emotionally."[33] She included facts about the Reach to Recovery Foundation, the nonprofit organization she created to support this work. The manual also outlined thirteen different exercises that helped restore movement to the arm after a mastectomy. Finally, it offered insight about clothing, bras, and fashion and how these shaped personal responses to a cancer diagnosis and a mastectomy.

Lasser started this grassroots program soon after her own breast cancer diagnosis. She felt lonely and isolated after her mastectomy. She asked physicians to allow her to speak to other women who had been recently treated for breast cancer. Although she faced resistance from some doctors who did not feel that a layperson should be meeting with a medical patient, other physicians supported her cause, put her in contact with patients, and publicized her efforts. Lasser cooperated with medical professionals and respected their authority. Yet in spite of this complicity and nonconfrontational manner, she made a significant impact on patients' lives and ushered in an era where breast cancer survivors learned that they were part of a larger community.

Lasser's husband funded the first publication of her manual, but the Reach to Recovery Foundation covered the cost of future editions. Many women wrote for copies, and Lasser reprinted it in 1954, 1955, and 1957. She revised and reprinted it in 1960 and again in 1963. By the 1960s this small organization, started by the activism of one woman, had expanded to include thousands of members in all fifty states. This network of women exchanged information about diagnosis, treatment, and recovery. Moreover, the group provided both emotional and physical advice on issues that cancer literature had previously ignored.[34]

Surgical operations for breast cancer varied according to the surgeon, but after a radical mastectomy most women lost full motion in their arm. Daily exercises helped restore movement to the arm and strengthened the remaining muscles. Lasser urged breast cancer survivors to exercise their arms regularly and recommended various movements that mirrored everyday activities. Hair brushing, paper crumbling, hanging clothes on a clothesline, opening window dressings, and an array of "household exercises," such as vacuuming and dusting, helped most women regain arm functions. Lasser also recommended specific exercises such as squeezing a rubber ball, walking arms up a wall, and rotating the shoulder. Lasser's therapeutic guidance supported the recommended medical treatment to restore arm movement after breast surgery. Much of this advice was gendered, linking women with domesticity and prioritizing the value of the physical body, but it created a dialogue that had previously been absent.[35]

Lasser always cooperated with the medical establishment and insisted that Reach to Recovery volunteers follow this lead. Volunteers only contacted patients after a physician's approval. Moreover, the manual consistently reminded readers to defer to their doctor's recommendation even if it differed from the Reach to Recovery advice. For instance, before describing the various rehabilitation exercises, Lasser wrote, "It is of the utmost importance that you follow your physician's directions carefully in undertaking any of the exercises which follow. He alone is qualified to tell you where you may begin, and how far you may go."[36] Even when emphasizing the value of artificial breast, the manual included the physician. "Just as soon as your doctor gives permission," the manual suggested, "arrange to be fitted with one of the many kinds of prosthetic devices which are available in almost all department stores and specialty shops."[37] Lasser further explained, "A prosthesis should do three things for a woman: first, give weight to the side of the operation, thus holding down the bra; second, go around a little on the side and on the top when necessary, thus helping to take the place of the lost muscles; third, give her back her figure. Unless it does all three, it is not fulfilling its purpose." The manual also included practical instruction for anchoring lightweight breast forms, creating fill-ins for depression areas in the arms and shoulders, adjusting straps to fit more properly, and caring for the skin. The booklet provided instructions for dyeing the conventional white cotton breast forms, supplied by the ACS, so that they matched the individual's skin color: "Dip the form cover in a strong brew of coffee or tea; if that doesn't darken it enough, use a good dye. In general the dye will not damage the form. You can also tint most breast forms the same way." Concerns such as matching the skin color of the prosthetic device to a woman's skin tone likely reflected both a concern for racial diversity and an awareness of the psychological import of the part. The closer its resemblance to a natural breast, the more likely a woman might imagine it as her own.[38]

In 1969 the ACS adopted Reach to Recovery. By then the women's organization had grown exponentially. By merging with the ACS, it gained formal organizational structure, administrative assistance, more volunteers, and access to financial support. It maintained the original framework established by Lasser that cooperated with physicians in an unchallenging and nonthreatening manner. Throughout the 1970s, the organization sent women who were recently diagnosed with breast cancer a "help packet," which contained a simple, temporary, foam breast pad. Reach to Recovery volunteers continued to visit women who had been recently treated for breast cancer, shared their personal experiences with the disease, and allowed patients to ask questions that they might only feel comfortable asking of someone who had experienced a similar diagnosis and operation.[39]

Influenced by cultural norms of the 1950s, the Reach to Recovery program reinforced gender standards that insisted on female standards of beauty and a dominant American culture of normalcy in bodies. Yet, it also legitimized the value of women's sharing knowledge with each other, discussing their bodies after mastectomy, and learning about the health consequences of cancer after diagnosis. Although far from political and rooted in one-on-one conversations, the emergence of this group in midcentury signified a small step toward political consciousness where women embodied their knowledge of breast cancer and shared it with one another. Equally significant, Reach to Recovery identified an expanding community of female cancer survivors, many of whom remained active in cancer awareness for the next several decades.

A Film Examines Mastectomy

In 1958 the Oregon Division of the ACS produced a twenty-one-minute film, *After Mastectomy*, that depicted many of the themes of the Reach to Recovery Program.[40] The film opens with a close-up of a woman, Kay Elliot, who has recently had a mastectomy. As Elliot gardens, she articulates her thoughts: "That Sylvia couldn't keep her eyes off of me. Trying to figure out which one was mine and which came from the emporium." By featuring Elliot in action, the film immediately demonstrated that mastectomy patients could resume "normal" lives soon after surgery. It also tapped into breast cancer survivors' anxiety regarding wearing a prosthesis and public reaction. The scene shifts to a flashback of Elliot's visit to the doctor's office and her first indication that she needed a mastectomy to treat her breast cancer, allowing the viewer to better contextualize her story.

Returning again to the present, Elliot stares at a photograph of her husband, anxious about his reaction as well. The narrator wonders, "How can a patient be helped from the fear, depression, and pain so normal during the first day or so following the removal of a breast?" Continually reinforcing gendered norms, the film portrays Kay Elliot as a domestic wife concerned about her husband. Going another step, the narrator suggests that unmarried women in particular worried about anyone (referring to potential husbands) caring for them after the surgery. Finally, the narrator acknowledges women's fear about whether the surgery removed all the cancer.

As the film proceeds, a nurse appears to console Elliot. Playing the role of feminine sympathy and support, the nurse asks, "Nothing helps more than putting your face on. Want some makeup?" Conflating the serious anxiety of a breast cancer diagnosis with the mundane details of grooming oneself allowed the audience to absorb the details of the film and the range of reactions that may accompany surgery. Likewise, it minimized the anxiety women likely experienced after cancer surgery. The nurse reminds Elliot that she needs to move her arm to restore mobility. Not atypical for the 1950s, the film relies on notions of female beauty once again, as the nurse demonstrates how applying makeup and brushing one's hair can serve as exercises that increase mobility.

Although the references to makeup seem trivial at first glance, they suggest a level of practicality in midcentury cancer awareness programs. Educational films, like their equivalent textual sources, wanted to teach patients without creating a paralyzing reaction to cancer. Informed by the ACS's support of aggressive treatment and eager to convince patients that radical mastectomy was a necessary procedure, the film and the ACS minimized the impact of mastectomy. Reach to Recovery responded to this tendency, in part, by acknowledging a web of fears that many recently diagnosed women shared. At second glance, the film moved beyond a surface discussion of grooming and female beauty standards. At the hospital, Elliot expresses her medical concerns to her doctor. She inquires about the results of the surgery and the chances that the cancer has spread. Her conversation reveals the details of her surgery (notably after the fact), celebrates the virtue of the radical mastectomy by positively portraying the removal of the pectoral muscles, and offers a hopeful prognosis, which the doctor attributes to her prompt and radical treatment.

Soon, the film features Elliot reading an ACS pamphlet, *Help Yourself to Recovery*, which listed arm and shoulder exercises for women who have had a mastectomy.[41] Similar to the *Reach to Recovery* manual and Kay's conversation with the nurse, this pamphlet relied on gendered assumptions for each description. It told women to hang clothes on a line, wash windows, and brush hair. Nodding toward the idea that mastectomy also involved issues of intimacy, the doctor explains to Kay's husband that the greatest thing he could do was to "let her know that his feelings, towards her as a husband, haven't changed." With such images of normalcy, the film addressed issues of body image, but it was uncompromising in its insistence that life could return to normal and the effects of surgery could and should be disguised. Women were encouraged to identify themselves as survivors in order to contribute to an awareness campaign based on the notion of cure, but this communal identity was not perceived as a threat the medical establishment or to the conventional standards advanced by the ACS.

Although *After Mastectomy* recognized a broad range of concerns, it claimed that women should overcome anxieties about mastectomy and breast cancer. Endorsing a simple outreach and educational program, the film claimed that most women would survive the surgery without significant consequences. "With the help from their doctors, nurses, and families," the film concludes, "the Kay Elliots of this world will recover with a few scars from their mild depressions and anxieties. There are others, however, who will be disturbed, even profoundly disturbed. These will need more time and help. Even to those with the greatest inner strength, appearance is important." Labeling women who failed to conform to this standard of quick recovery as "profoundly disturbed," the film allowed for no cultural representation of women who challenged conventional treatment. Moreover, the messages of the film reinforced many common patterns evident in the textual discourse of popular journals. By focusing on the restoration of the body and breast and prioritizing the importance of physical appearance, these educational programs introduced a superficial discussion of breast cancer survival into popular American culture.

In the final scenes of the film, the nurse teaches Elliot how to insert cotton into her bra to give the appearance of a breast. "I've got cotton," the nurse says, "Let's see what we can do to fool the public." A Reach to Recovery volunteer, Mrs. Evans, comes in to show Elliot her prosthetic breast and reminds Elliot to shop until she could find one that really fit. Evans bluntly states, there is "nothing easy about readjusting after the shock of losing a breast." The film concludes with an image that suggests successful rehabilitation, Elliot triumphantly throwing a tennis ball.

Like the creation of Reach to Recovery and its message of cure and normalcy, this film represented a departure in cancer awareness programming. Popular knowledge about cancer had moved beyond simple messages of early detection and reminders such as "do not delay."[42] Throughout the second half of the century, cancer education material had begun to explicitly address issues of treatment and the consequences of cancer surgery. American women learned details about breast cancer treatment, and films and education programs recognized a community of survivors.

The content of these messages and the historical circumstances in which they emerged undermined the potential for community and group formation. Although breast cancer survivors shared an identity, the identity remained largely apolitical, defined by individual concerns. Within the next two decades, however, during a period of social unrest and political activism, the community that failed to transform breast cancer care at midcentury would insist on immediate transformation.

By the late 1950s women had also learned that their compliance with cancer guidelines would include annual screenings that employed modern technology. The faith in science and technology that accompanied the end of World War II contributed to emerging hopes that better cancer screening would facilitate cancer cures. Support for technological solutions had created funding for Dr. Papanicolaou's vaginal smear, and by the late 1950s the ACS had begun promotion of its first program for mass cancer screening.

Publicity for the Pap Smear

After more than a decade of local studies that had begun in the late 1940s, the national society felt that it could finally provide the testing centers and equipment necessary to screen all women in the United States for cervical cancer. When the ACS launched its cervical cancer screening program in 1957, it coordinated its efforts with physician groups, women's groups, and medical centers. It also outlined an educational agenda that offered little departure from its earlier practice. Namely, although cancer screening was a revolutionary and controversial breakthrough, it was presented to the public as part of a continuum in early detection practices. It insisted that women must detect cancer early for cancer cures to be effective.

The 1957 uterine/cervical cancer screening campaign incorporated a "ten-step plan," which reflected the deliberateness associated with this cancer awareness effort. Unlike early efforts that focused primarily on teaching women about the value of early detection, this program included comprehensive planning that coordinated public awareness, medical education, and technological preparedness. As the ACS outlined, cervical cancer awareness needed to include:

1. Planning
2. Seeking support of pathologists
3. Enlisting endorsement of professional societies
4. Recruiting and training cytotechnicians
5. Securing adequate laboratory facilities
6. Informing physicians of the program
7. Beginning the public education campaign
8. Establishing continuity of examination
9. Preserving the doctor-patient relationship
10. Making the program self-supporting

More so than any other early detection program to date, this program required professional participation and training. Throughout the first half of the century, laywomen had been able to effectively promulgate the message of early detection. Now, however, physicians needed to directly participate in early detection promotion by informing their female patients about this screening tool, planning for its implementation, and carrying out the goals outlined by the ACS.[43]

Barriers to universal screening proved ubiquitous. Many medical professionals questioned the practical application of the smear, while others argued about the usefulness of the exam and how often it should be conducted. Between 1960 and 1965 debates about the recommended frequency of the exam most often centered on the patient's age. Although some physicians believed that only women over the age of thirty needed to be tested, others recommended routine vaginal smears for younger women.[44] In a debate that foreshadowed contemporary discussions about mammography, the vaginal smear created intense conflict as health activists created a protocol meant to serve all women.

The ACS sponsored educational campaigns that taught women about the Pap smear. It produced posters and pamphlets, and it encouraged popular periodicals to describe the procedure. It also created the film *Time and Two Women*, which compared two women's experiences with uterine (cervical) cancer.[45] Like early twentieth-century narratives, this film relied on a dichotomy whereby one woman followed early detection advice and survived cancer, while her counterpart failed to adhere to this advice and died. The film reflected the pervasiveness of the morality tale in cancer awareness that insisted that patient compliance with medical advice ensured healthy outcomes. The release of this film marked the start of a national education effort to promote cancer screening.

Three years after the release of *Time and Two Women*, the American Cancer Society launched its second major public relations effort to promote cervical cancer screening. In 1960 it started the "Conquer Uterine Cancer" program with an immediate goal of doubling the number of women who had periodic uterine cancer exams from 5 million to 10 million. Although the ACS hoped that ultimately all physicians would include routine Pap smears in annual physical exams for women, in 1960 this modest goal reflected the hurdle of normalizing the exam so that it could gradually be incorporated into routine preventive practices in women's health. As in its 1930s recruitment drive for the Women's Field Army, the ACS invited the General Federation of Women's Clubs (GFWC) to join its program. The GFWC readily agreed, and in 1961 the ACS reported that 3,500 women's organizations affiliated with the GFWC were "actively participating, with some reporting the full cooperation of their membership."[46]

Unlike female cancer awareness programs in the 1930s, 1940s, and 1950s, the "Conquer Uterine Cancer" program appealed to racially and ethnically diverse audiences. For instance, in 1961 the ACS produced a special Spanish-language version of *Time and Two Women*.[47]

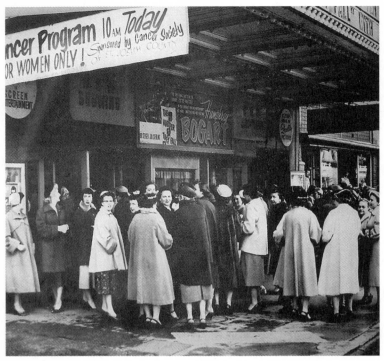

As the 2,500-person theater filled, hundreds of women were turned away from this cancer program in South Bend, Indiana, in 1957. (Courtesy of American Cancer Society)

Two years later, it recruited three national women's organizations unaffiliated with the GFWC to join the program—the National Council of Negro Women (NCNW), the National Council of Catholic Women, and Pilot Club International. The NCNW soon launched its own "CON-QUER UTERINE CANCER NOW: An American Cancer Society Project in Cooperation with the National Council of Negro Women."[48]

In January 1963 NCNW president Dorothy I. Height wrote to all NCNW affiliate presidents.[49] Describing the "CONQUER UTERINE CAN-CER NOW" campaign as a "unique" and "life-saving" program, she expressed her full support for this cooperative effort. Height assured her colleagues of the ACS's commitment to the program and encouraged all chapters to support it. She concluded her letter in a spirited tone: "Let's show the world what an organization of public-spirited women, as represented in our Council's membership, can do when presented with such a challenge!" The ACS offered publicity, pamphlets, fact sheets, speech outlines, and press releases to the NCNW. In addition, it promised to organize viewings of *Time and Two Women*. To be sure, *Time and Two Women* featured an all-white cast. Although the ACS welcomed the NCNW as a way to target African American female audiences, it did not create alternative publications or films specifically for this audience. Height's cooperation with the ACS and her willingness to distribute this film likely reflect the limited resources for African American health activists in the 1960s and her eagerness to address the high rate of uterine cancer in the African American female population.[50]

A few months later Estelle Osbourne, a leader in the NCNW, agreed to serve as national chair of the NCNW's cancer awareness program. Writing to the presidents of the national organizations in the NCNW, Osbourne explained the program's objective: "To reach as many Negro women as we possibly can—through our organizations and then within the communities in which we live—to urge that they begin a life-long habit of annual physical checkups including a 'Pap' test." Emphasizing that black women died from uterine cancer at twice the rate of white women, Osbourne encouraged every black woman to join this effort. She also urged chapters to record the number of women who participated in the program, declaring it a "history-making project" that would reduce the number of black women who died from uterine cancer. In addition to providing statistical data, organizers anticipated greater local cooperation if goals could be set and participation tracked.[51]

Literature and programs for white audiences also encouraged the adoption of routine Pap smears. Throughout the 1960s white women's clubs continued to screen *Time and Two Women* and then afterward host medical specialists who could answer questions about cancer. The efforts to encourage Pap smears paralleled the efforts to encourage breast self-exams, with the film *Time and Two Women* serving a similar function as the film *The Breast Self-Examination*.

The campaigns helped to inform women about cervical cancer screening. A 1961 Gallup Poll recorded that 30 percent of American women had had the Pap test at least once. Two years later, the figure was 48 percent. Moreover, by 1964, 77 percent of women had heard of the test. The ACS hoped to continue to increase these percentages. In particular, it wanted to educate women who had never heard of the Pap smear. As the ACS explained, "A prime target here is the non-white segment of the population, where the death rate from uterine cancer is more than twice that of white females." Another Gallup Poll confirmed this observation. Although 52 percent of white women had had a Pap smear in 1963, only 22 percent of black women had a Pap smear.[52]

In the mid-1960s the American Cancer Society declared that "the most encouraging story is that for cancer of the cervix of the uterus."[53] The smear represented a new frontier in effective early detection. Celebrating this project, the ACS designed an exhibit for the Hall of Science at the 1964 New York World's Fair that featured the story of the Pap test, the ACS's support for it, and the subsequent decline in deaths from uterine cancer. The exhibit stimulated "the interest of young visitors in research careers" while at the same time helping "women realize the importance of the test as a life-saving potential in their own lives."[54] As visitors entered the World's Fair, they were surrounded by material artifacts meant to suggest the wonders of modernity; for cancer advocates of the 1960s, the Pap smear represented modern science's successful efforts at fighting cancer.

In 1970 the ACS released another educational film focused on uterine cancer. *It's Up To You*, a thirteen-minute color film, stressed the importance of annual Pap smears.[55] Like many early films produced by the ACS, the opening scene pans the faces of a group of women gathered to hear a medical lecture. However, unlike early films, which usually featured an all-white cast, this one included a more racially diverse group of women. For example, at one point, the camera focuses on a young white mother, a black grandmother, and a middle-aged white teacher. Although the cast still seemed dominated by middle-class women, the racial diversity reflected the increased attention of the ACS on the need to depict a more representative population. The speaker, a male white doctor, offers a short talk about the importance of annual physical exams that should include a Pap smear.

After the meeting, at a reception in the cafeteria, a woman asks the doctor about the procedural steps involved in a Pap smear. The female audience attentively listens to his answer. The audience learns that the test is quick and could be performed in gynecology clinics, private offices, or hospitals (although a hospital visit was not necessary). A specialist would insert a speculum into the vagina, scrape cells from the neck of the cervix, and then smear these cells onto a slide. The doctor assures the audience that the test is not painful. He stresses that this exam could diagnose cells in their precancerous stage. Confidently, he claims that if every woman would visit a doctor every year for a pelvic exam and Pap smear, then there would be a good chance of total eradication of cervical cancer.

Finally, the film traces one woman's experience with the Pap smear. Relying on gendered notions of motherhood, the woman's comments indicate that her devotion to her family inspired her to have the Pap smear. She describes the duty of motherhood as twofold: caring for the family's health and protecting herself from cancer and death. Moreover, she recalls that her mother had died from cancer, and she expresses concern about her increased risk for cancer due to genetics.

The audience next hears about this woman's positive experience in the physician's office. When she visited the doctor, he explained the procedure to her. He then demonstrated it on a plastic model before performing it on her. Afterward, the woman declared that the exam was painless. In the final film sequence, she carries her groceries with a huge smile—"A year without fear and worry." The narrator chimes in as the voice of medical authority: "We have the knowledge, the rest is up to you."

The title and the closing dialogue of *It's Up to You* indicate that cancer awareness programs continued to insist that women recognize cancer in its earliest stage. Even in the midst of celebrating cellular studies that could reveal precancerous cells—studies that took place inside hospital laboratories outside of the domain of the patient's control—the popular messages of early detection continued to imply that women's individual behavior contributed to cancer outcomes. As had been stated for decades, early detection would lead to a cure, while procrastination could lead to death. Although intended to improve patient compliance, this message had the unintended consequences of blaming the victim and deflecting public dialogue about contributing factors to cancer, the quality of life after diagnosis, and the acceptance of death when diagnosed with one of the leading causes of death in the United States.

Although the Pap smear reinforced the rhetoric of early detection that had defined cancer awareness since 1913, the cells revealed "cancer in situ," which were precancerous cells. Distinct from the breast self-examination, which might reveal a cancer tumor, the vaginal smear had far-reaching potential as a preventive exam. Cancer in situ cells could be removed before they became cancerous. Although this distinction is clear and significant, popular cancer discourse of the late 1960s and 1970s often conflated cancer screening to indicate precancerous cells and early cancer detection.[56] This tendency inflated the value of the breast self-examination and implied that breast cancer could be detected at an equally early stage. The vaginal smear's success served to validate decades of early detection rhetoric that continued to shift blame to the victim for late diagnosis.[57]

Early cancer awareness campaigns that encouraged women to embrace this technology are only one part of the broader story of the history of the Pap smear. As sociologists Monica Casper and Adele Clarke have persuasively demonstrated, the successful implementation of the Pap smear was due to several converging factors. The test succeeded because it could be completed by technicians, who could be paid as skilled laborers, thus avoiding the higher salaries of medical professionals. Mass screening was accomplished in part by hiring women, who were typically paid lower wages, to read thousands of slides per week. Casper and Clarke's work exposes the nuances that surrounded the implementation of this tool and its practicality for mass screening.[58]

Local Initiatives: Cedar Rapids, Iowa

Although popular discussions of cancer were expanded after World War II to consider treatment protocol and patient experiences after cancer treatment, local studies reveal how these changes occurred over time and were influenced by regional concerns. On a local level, some physicians had long discussed treatment protocol with patients and altered treatment to better serve their needs. One such example occurred in Cedar Rapids, Iowa, where a physician's records reveal that frequent interaction with female patients and women's groups influenced his protocol. A closer look at his involvement in cancer awareness indicates the cooperation that sometimes emerged between cancer physicians and cancer educators. Between 1920 and the 1950s, Arthur Erskine questioned the merits of radical surgery and ushered in effective Pap smear screening in a rural community.

Activists in Iowa, one of the first states to sponsor radio programs on breast and uterine cancer awareness, host films of the breast self-examination, and study the effects of the Pap smear, achieved many of the ACS's national education and research goals. Local physician Arthur Erskine contributed to many of these programs, and his career offers a lens through which we can examine the effective liaisons that formed between female educators and a male physician dedicated to cancer awareness. Like that of many local initiatives, the success of Iowa's female cancer awareness programs was due to the combined efforts of female activists who facilitated awareness sessions and the male doctors who often served as ACS "experts." Moreover, the cooperation that emerged between Erskine and the female educators in this midwestern state fostered a dialogue that enabled the transfer of medical knowledge from professional to lay audiences.

Arthur Wright Erskine graduated from the Baltimore Medical College in 1908. After an internship in Baltimore, graduate work at John

Hopkins University, and a brief residency in Pennsylvania, he settled in Cedar Rapids, Iowa in 1912. A specialist in radiology, he created x-ray departments at several Cedar Rapids hospitals and gained an international reputation for his work in this field over the next forty years. Unaffiliated with a major research institution, Erskine conducted his experiments, which included extensive studies on x-ray treatment for cervical cancer, at the local Coe College physics laboratory. In 1931 he published his first authoritative work, *Practical x-Ray Treatment.*[59]

During the early decades of his career (1903–25), Erskine studied the power, direction, and strength of various forms of light. Fascinated by its potential as a medical tool, he worked to standardize the field of radiology and create a unit of measurement recognized across international boundaries. Erskine believed radiology could become a more effective adjuvant cancer therapy and could also serve as the primary treatment for cancers inaccessible by surgery.[60]

Erskine's experiences with breast and uterine cancer informed much of his research. He recorded success with radiation treatment in an era when most medical professionals focused on surgical solutions to cancer, and he advocated aggressive radiation treatment as a tool for curing breast and uterine cancers (instead of aggressive surgery), believing the benefits of this treatment outweighed any potential risks. As he explained, "I am one of those who believes that the radical operation for cancer of the breast, with block dissection of the axilla, might well be abandoned because it is unnecessary in the early cases and futile in the late ones." Erskine argued that intense radiation killed the cancer cells that surgery failed to remove. He criticized the radical, Halsted mastectomy as the standard treatment for breast cancer, and although he did not define a systemic behavior of cancer, he advocated a therapy based on it. Further, he urged physicians to use routine, postoperative x-ray treatment for all breast cancers as a way to avoid metastasis.[61]

Committed to early detection of cancer, Erskine actively participated in the ASCC. He served on Iowa's WFA executive committee and routinely spoke to women's clubs throughout the state. As his nurse of six years, Bernice Prunskunas, recalled, Erskine spent time with his patients, encouraged them, and adjusted his research/treatment in response to patient experiences. As his obituary surmised, "Probably no one knows any more about cancer than Arthur Erskine did, but he was never hesitant to admit the great limitations of that knowledge and never too busy to listen to anybody with an idea that might conceivably hold a clue to the answers neither he nor anyone could give."[62] Familiar with patient reticence to seek treatment, Erskine suggested that surgeons offer women alternative choices of treatment. As he explained in 1922, "A conservative plan of treatment will reduce the immediate operative mortality and tend to remove the fear of crippling operation from the minds of the laity, and induce them to submit to operation earlier in the course of their disease."[63]

Erskine's critiques of radical mastectomy stemmed from his concern about the extensive nature of Halsted's methods. Although Erskine placed male physicians in a hierarchical position where they might induce women to "submit," his views offered women a limited form of agency and insisted that physicians needed to respond to patients' concerns. It seems that his female audiences and patients convinced him that women delayed treatment because they dreaded the effects of surgery. Erskine recognized that treatment needed to be evaluated within the context of patient experience and therefore suggested that physicians offer conservative surgical treatment options as a way to lessen the dread and increase compliance with suggested guidelines of prompt medical attention.[64]

Many women who had a radical mastectomy lost the full motion of their arm, suffered from lymphedema or swelling of the arm, and experienced pain after the surgery. Recognizing these patterns, Erskine urged women to question the worthiness of radical surgery. He treated women's medical concerns as legitimate subjects, rather than trying to coerce women with strong medical advice.[65] He also refuted the notion that women were to blame for late diagnosis. Instead, he questioned the physician's role: "The principal reason for the present disgraceful mortality rate in cancer of the breast is delay. We, as physicians, might now be more usefully employed in devising methods of avoiding or reducing this dangerous delay than in perfecting the technical details of our own art."[66] Erskine believed that invasive and painful treatment led some women to resist early detection and treatment. Although a seemingly simple observation, his attention to female patient experiences was extraordinary in both midcentury Iowa and within the broader agenda of cancer awareness. Likewise, his critique of radical surgery proved farsighted. As he wrote, "I believe that little is gained by surgical invasion of the axilla, and that these patients will have a longer and more comfortable life if the primary tumor only be excised and x-rays depended upon to control the axillary, supra-clavicular, and mediastinal extensions."[67]

Erskine's research on radiation as a treatment for breast, cervical, and uterine cancers influenced the leadership roles he assumed in Iowa Cancer Efforts, the American Society for the Control of Cancer, and the American Cancer Society. As early as 1935, Erskine served as one of three members of an Iowa Cancer Committee (ICC) and encouraged layperson education as one of its primary objectives. He cooperated with women who organized cancer lectures and presentations and urged female cancer advocates to spread the message of early detection far and wide, implying that the full potential of early detection would only be realized with their participation. Similar to national trends of female volunteerism, women promoted cancer awareness in this midwestern state by recruiting audiences, arranging convenient meeting places, and confirming speakers such as Erskine.

When Erskine spoke to audiences, often entirely female audiences, he stressed the value of early detection. Joining a team of medical volunteers from the Iowa State Medical Society and the ICC who toured throughout Iowa to lecture on the topic of cancer and early detection, he participated in numerous women's gatherings designed to promote cancer education. Erskine's lecturing schedule in the mid-1930s included meetings with the Women's Clubs of Des Moines, the Women's Auxiliary to the County Medical Society (an organization of doctors' wives), the Convention of Federated Women's Clubs, and to the Women's Clubs in Tipton. He asked female audiences to join in cancer education with the same fervor that they had brought to the tuberculosis movement. "The commonest site of cancer in women is the uterus," he argued. "Its warning is an unusual discharge, bloody or watery which may be a mere spotting or may take the form of a hemorrhage. You must teach all women that any discharge after the menopause calls for an immediate visit to the doctor, and a thorough investigation to find out that it is or is not cancer." He similarly explained, "One sentence tells you all you need to know about cancer of the breast. The finding of a painless lump in the breast should send a woman galloping to her physician."[68] His rhetoric thus echoed the standard messages of the ASCC, and as his reference to "galloping" suggests, he also stressed the need to seek medical consultation immediately at the first indication of cancer.

The Women's Field Army organized in Cedar Rapids in 1937. The Cedar Rapids WFA quickly arranged a state tour for Erskine, who had volunteered to be one of its medical speakers, and urged that he talk about cancers specific to women.[69] Following WFA guidelines, Erskine emphasized female susceptibility to cancer, impressed upon his audiences that early cancers responded to treatment, and insisted that doctors could cure cancer if diagnosis occurred in the early stages of the disease. In addition to his speaking role, Erskine served on the Iowa WFA executive committee.[70]

The WFA also secured radio time at a time when some radio programs hesitated to say the word "cancer" on the air. Working with station managers, women convinced those who controlled the local radio stations to share radio space for this worthwhile cause. Erskine's radio addresses reflected the latitude that WFA volunteers ensured. In "Cancer Control," Erskine bluntly explained, "The breast is an accessible organ and can be felt easily. When a woman feels a lump in her breast she should consult a physician immediately." He similarly described the difficulty of treating late-stage uterine cancer: "Too often women come in, stating they have had abnormal bleeding for several months and feel it a normal thing for them during the change of life. This erroneous idea causes many women to seek aid late."[71]

The Iowa WFA, female activists, and Erskine expressed concern about teaching female cancer awareness in rural areas, with scattered populations of women. Unlike urban areas, Erskine argued, "there are geographic, economic, and perhaps psychological conditions in our state, and in other rural states" that might interfere with early detection efforts.[72] Iowa cancer activists recognized that many people would not want to travel to remote urban cancer centers for treatment: "They get homesick and discouraged and abandon treatment before they should. In practice, therefore, the great majority of patients with cancer must now, and for some time to come, be treated in or near their own communities. We must do the best we can with what we have." Through a medical lens, Erskine realized that local treatment facilities might be inferior to centralized, better-equipped urban centers, but he also considered the unique behavioral tendencies of his target population. Less superior treatment was better than no treatment. "If we were invariably to insist upon institutional treatment," Erskine posited, "the death rate would be likely to rise instead of fall."[73] As these speeches illustrate, Erskine relied on the female volunteers of the WFA to orchestrate the spreading of his message; he even adopted their rhetoric prioritizing early detection. Nevertheless, his local experience led him to insist that treatment procedures respond to the specific needs of their recipients.

His speeches to colleagues suggest the ways that he continued to challenge the primacy of radical surgery. Reiterating points he made in medical journals in the 1920s and 1930s, he asked colleagues in greater Philadelphia in the early 1940s, "Why must we always insist upon doing the best possible thing, theoretically, for each patient, when too often our insistence means that nothing will be or can be done? The patient with early cancer of the breast who is willing to submit to a simple mammectomy but refuses or postpones a radical operation because she fears it may spread the disease or cripple her is just as dead as if we had exhausted all the skill and science at our command and still had failed." After countless discussions at women's clubs and years of interactions with women seeking treatment for cancer, he was convinced that many patients delayed treatment because they feared it, suspected it would not work, or believed such severe treatment was unwarranted. In case his message was unclear, or unconvincing, he described a parallel scenario: "When everyone believed that the best treatment for cancer of the lip [was] excision of the lesion with radical dissection of the glands of the neck, the death rate was high, not because the treatment was bad, it was very good, but because to the patients it seemed too extensive, too mutilating, too expensive, too time-consuming for what seemed to them to be such an insignificant disease. It was not until simpler, less expensive, locally destructive methods were accepted and applied that any real progress was made in reducing the death rate."[74]

At the same time, the Iowa chapter of the ACS devoted much attention to female cancers.[75] In 1950–51 the speaker's bureau concentrated on showing *The Breast Self-Examination* to the women of the state. The Iowa chapter purchased seventy-seven prints of the film, showed it 2,400 times in 1951, and estimated that 104,000 women in Iowa had seen it. Dr. E. G. Zimmerer coordinated the film project, described as "the greatest educational project in our history—the saturation of Iowa with showings of the film *Breast Self-Examination*." Local activists, usually women and volunteers, recognized a need to inform their communities and organized multiple programs. In addition to film screenings, Iowa newspapers donated nearly 65,000 column inches to cancer information and 5,000 column inches of advertising space. Radio stations donated 2,400 quarter-hour programs.[76]

Such local commitment, experience, and activism, coupled with women's traditional philanthropy, made the Iowa ACS a breeding ground for new programs. While the national ACS debated the best way to proceed with the vaginal smear as a screening tool for the population at large, locally the Iowa ACS embarked on a small and specific study that would determine the test's effect in this community. Hester Sinclair donated $5,000 to the Iowa ACS, and this money supported the "Papanicolaou Test in the Cancer Control Program."[77]

It was Erskine who first convinced the Iowa ACS to subsidize a local study of the Pap smear. The ACS donated $12,000 to the program, which started in 1947 when personnel at the Gynecology Department of the State University of Iowa City performed vaginal smears on all women over thirty years of age who were admitted to the hospital. In addition, physicians performed vaginal smears on all female residents of the two state mental hospitals. Clinicians collected a total of 5,214 smears and from these diagnosed 200 cancer cases.[78]

By 1948, preliminary results of the Iowa study confirmed the effectiveness of the Pap smear as an effective screening tool. Cancer activists in Cedar Rapids proposed an expansion of the Pap study to include routine tests in both Cedar Rapids hospitals and private offices in the area. Vaginal smears could be collected in any location, cells could be fixed to slides there, and then slides could be transported to a central cytology lab in Iowa City for a final reading.[79] The Iowa ACS approved the proposal, and in 1948 Cedar Rapids became the first city in Iowa, and one of the first cities in the United States, to begin mass screening of women using Pap smears.[80] Erskine served as one of the organizers of this study that set an ambitious goal: testing every woman over the age of thirty in Cedar Rapids in any medical facility. Testing occurred in private physician offices as well as hospital laboratories. National, state, and local ACS funds paid for the bulk of the lab equipment and a full-time staff member. The Linn County Medical Society asked its members to waive their usual fee to ensure that all women could afford the exam. Its members agreed, and women paid one dollar to cover the lab costs of the test.[81]

The Iowa study would ultimately serve as a model for a national program for cervical cancer screening. Erskine anticipated success in the cervical cancer detection program in part because of his intense devotion to early detection and subsequent treatment. As he told Hester Sinclair, "In the first 165 cases examined three very early cancers were found and the patients were cured." Hoping women would continue to donate funds to cancer research, he added a personal message: "This, incidentally, was about the amount of work your contribution paid for."[82]

The dedication to the Pap smear studies reflected the optimism evident since 1913 that early detection would allow for more effective control of cancer. It also foretold the new emphasis on scientific research. As the Iowa research statement read in the early 1950s:

Iowans have faith in scientific research as a primary means of solving the problem of cancer. A recent survey showed that contributors to the ACS believed so strongly in research that they rated it as somewhat more important than the education of the public to detect cancer's danger signals and to seek prompt treatment. Historically it has always been the role of volunteers to take the initiative and provide the inspiration for attacking a social problem such as cancer. Although the division's means were limited, it was determined that cancer research should be developed and encouraged in Iowa so as to stimulate general action on the part of the state and federal agencies.[83]

Cancer education goals required cooperation between the local educators, who were primarily female, and local medical experts, who were primarily male. Female volunteers readily adopted the rhetoric of early detection endorsed by professionals such as Erskine. Yet awareness efforts throughout Iowa reflected the complicated relationship that emerged between patients, educators, and physicians. As Erskine's story reveals, physicians, female volunteers, and audiences all learned more about cancer during education and awareness programs. In these sessions, women heard information about common cancer symptoms, and physicians heard women express their fears and concerns about cancer. Many women who organized cancer awareness programs invited female audiences to share their fears and concerns about modern cancer treatment. When women facilitated such dialogue, physicians such as Erskine gained a keener appreciation of the patient experience. Erskine ultimately reconsidered the merits of surgery, radiation, and x-ray vis-à-vis the patient experience. As a result, he came to criticize medical protocols that created undue fear.[84] Although his most vocal critique of radical surgery was often directed at a professional audience, his cooperation with lay populations, the ACS, and its female audiences informed his views.

Erskine's devotion to public education continued throughout his life. In 1937 he published a small pamphlet, *Cancer: A Manual for the Public*. Continuously revised and expanded, by the early 1950s this instructive manual included over fifty pages of cancer information written for a public audience. As Erskine wrote, "We have no constructive cures for cancer. . . . We hope that eventually some such constructive cure will be found, but at present the only effective methods of curing cancer are destructive."[85]

To medical professionals, Erskine offered three suggestions. First, he urged physicians to consider replacing radical mastectomy with a simple mastectomy. Next, he believed that "a more pessimistic attitude with the patients who already have metastases" could serve patients more than misinformation or false hopes. Finally, he hoped that scientific discourse might recognize its limits and faults without decreasing its legitimacy. As one example, he noted the difficulty of distinguishing between malignant and benign tumors.[86]

His first suggestion reflected his concern about a medical profession that dismissed alternative therapy and less aggressive treatments. He instead recognized the voice of patients when he told colleagues, "These women fear the radical operation, and many of them believe that it may spread the disease, or cripple them."[87] His next suggestion about metastases urged physicians to limit false optimism and share the reality of a diagnosis with their patients. His third suggestion admitted to uncertainty and condoned preventive mastectomy (in cases of doubt he advocated surgery), when scientific results remained vague.

Local efforts in Iowa suggest some of the ways that female activists and male professionals interacted. The programs also suggest that female patients who discussed their diagnosis, either individually with physicians, family, or friends, or more publicly through printed narratives, expanded the lay conversations of cancer in the postwar years. Acknowledgement of the uncertainty in cancer studies, the effects of treatment, and the controversies in adjuvant therapy reflected the complicated state of cancer and cancer awareness.

Communities throughout the United States continued to learn

about early detection, and educators cultivated a sense of hope and optimism. Within this context, local groups such as the ICC could adopt the educational tools of the ACS (pamphlets, films, and more) and share them with audiences in a manner that would be appropriate for each specific locality. Local considerations shaped the educational agenda and sometimes, as in the case of Cedar Rapids, created an environment where physicians learned from their patients and questioned conventional medical wisdom. In spite of this possibility, the national message of early detection was reinforced in many localities, and the sense that individuals bore responsibility for cancer prevention resonated loudly. Although education proved useful, its insistence that women could detect cancer early implied that women who failed to discover cancer in its earliest stage bore some culpability for their diagnosis.

Erskine published throughout his career, and his work has been archived by the Grand Masonic Lodge of Cedar Rapids. Although these documents reflect the story of one physician in a midwestern city, it is likely that other physicians throughout the country shared some of his concerns and practices. Also, the small and rural population of Cedar Rapids created an intimate network of volunteers, patients, physicians, friends, and family that may have fostered a more nuanced discussion of cancer, its impact, and the consequences of cancer treatment.

By midcentury, the majority of medical professionals, as well as the majority of Americans who were informed about cancer, believed that early and aggressive treatment for cancer offered the best possibility for a cure. As testament to the educational campaign spearheaded by the ACS, few imagined that cancer treatment could be scaled back or that women could have time to contemplate a diagnosis before surgery. For half a century the ACS has been repeating messages of early detection and prompt treatment, emphasizing the significance of time and insisting on deference to medical authority. Yet, medical opinions divided in the 1950s and 1960s, and dissenting voices challenged the very premise of popular knowledge about cancer.[88]

Conclusion

The nature of cancer awareness changed in midcentury. Women continued to contribute to educational initiatives, yet the messages that they spread expanded in new and interesting directions. First, the euphoria of postwar society and its faith in science and technology fostered optimism about cancer screening technology for women. In spite of the complications associated with this project, including its cost and effectiveness, many cancer advocates embraced the idea of screening for earlier diagnosis. Second, the discussion of cancer expanded to include details about treatment and post-operative concerns. Clearly, knowledge is power and patients were gradually accumulating more and more information about their diagnosis. However, at the same time that the discussions of post-operative concerns appeared in popular narratives, concerted efforts to encourage prosthesis appeared. The attention to prosthesis in the postwar era reflected the emphasis on female figures and beauty in midcentury. Cancer awareness advocates clung strongly to notions of normal appearance as healing processes in a very complicated illness.

The formal network of breast cancer survivors that started to form in 1954 under the guidance of Terese Lasser used their common experience of breast cancer to teach each other about recovery, both physical and emotional. Reach to Recovery offered a precursor and hinted at ideas that would later become essential to the women's health movement. Women learned about their bodies and discussed their common experiences in the medical system. They valued their experiential knowledge, often more than medical knowledge, and learned rehabilitation skills from each other. Although many conversations took place individually, among survivors, the volunteers working for Reach to Recovery created a community of women who had gradually begun to insert survivor's voices into a medical system that often deprived them of such a position and improved many women's experience in the medical system by doing so.

5

Screening Technology, Feminist
Health Movement, Cancer Critics

In the final decades of the twentieth century, women ushered
in major changes in American culture and gender relations
in U.S. society. Several trends contributed to these transformations, which directed critical attention to issues of women
and health. Most influential, the feminist health movement
insisted that women's voices and experiences gain more merit
in medical evaluations and treatment decisions. In addition,
unintended publicity, generated by First Lady Betty Ford and
vice presidential wife Happy Rockefeller, trained the focus
of public discourse and media attention on breast cancer.[1]
As a second screening technology, mammography, emerged
for women, debates about the efficacy and cost of screening
for breast cancer surfaced in public discussions.[2] Finally, the
creation of alternative cancer organizations, from 1970s organizations such as Y-ME to political organizations of the 1990s
such as the National Breast Cancer Coalition, rivaled the monopoly of the American Cancer Society (ACS) with its philanthropic strategies and successful publicity.[3] By the end of
the twentieth century, women's cancers were entrenched in
dominant American culture. As Barbara Ehrenreich noted in
2001, "it's the biggest disease on the cultural map, bigger than
AIDS, cystic fibrosis, or spinal injury, bigger even than those
more prolific killers of women—heart disease, lung cancer,
and stroke."[4]

This chapter explores the emergence of these cultural shifts, which introduced a political dimension to breast cancer awareness and recognized women's agency and influence in cancer policy. Beginning with the publicity generated by Betty Ford's breast cancer diagnosis, following with the subsequent mammography debates of the 1970s, and concluding with an analysis of the influence of women's health activists, this chapter describes a historical departure in cancer awareness that occurred in the final three decades of the twentieth century. Although the messages of early detection continued to resonate, and women's clubs and organizations continued to engage in cancer awareness, the rhetoric of women and cancer became imbued with a political and influential edge that informed public policy.

Betty Ford and Breast Cancer in the 1970s

In September 1974, a few months after Gerald Ford became president of the United States, fifty-six-year-old First Lady Betty Ford went to the Bethesda Naval Hospital for a routine gynecological examination. The physician noticed an abnormal lump in her breast, and Betty Ford scheduled a biopsy for two days later. The First Lady immediately decided that the American public should know about her health status and directed the White House to release a public statement.[5] Soon after she entered the hospital on Friday night, the White House announced, "Mrs. Betty Ford was examined at Bethesda Naval Hospital on Thursday morning for a regular medical check-up. During the process of that examination, a small nodule was detected in her right breast. After further medical consultation, it was recommended that the nodule be surgically removed and a biopsy be performed to determine whether it was benign or malignant. . . . Should it prove malignant, surgery would be performed to remove the right breast."[6]

Ford's biopsy and subsequent modified radical mastectomy riveted the American public. Although cancer education had been widespread for over half a century, the recent wave of notable American women publicizing a breast cancer diagnosis attracted the media's attention. Marvella Bayh, the wife of Senator Birch Bayh, announced her diagnosis in 1971, Shirley Temple Black announced her diagnosis in 1972, and Ford insisted that the public hear about her diagnosis in 1974.[7] As Ford later recalled: "As I look back, I am very pleased that when my breast cancer was detected in 1974, my family and I decided to make public my surgery. I knew it was going to be a shocking announcement to the news media, but I had no idea that over the years my decision would provide an awareness that would save the lives of many women. Through this awareness, women have realized the importance of early detection of breast cancer. I am happy I was able to be part of this realization."[8]

Betty Ford's announcement directed an unprecedented level of attention to breast cancer in the mid-1970s. First, early detection education programs, most evident among women's clubs, in women's magazines, or in programs orchestrated by the ACS, had never captured the co-ed audience that Ford's diagnosis did. Second, a political figure of such stature had never spoken about the disease so publicly, and newspapers and the media directed enormous coverage to this case of breast cancer.[9] Finally, her diagnosis coincided with mammography trials, sparking public interest in screening technology, and especially in the recently launched Breast Cancer Detection Demonstration Project (BCDDP), cosponsored by the American Cancer Society and the National Cancer Institute (NCI). After Ford's diagnosis, the public engaged in greater dialogue about mammography, and many women sought access to mammography screening at BCDDP centers.[10]

Ford's case offers a framework for examining shifts in cancer awareness during the 1970s for two reasons in particular. The publicity that she directed to her case of breast cancer contributed to changing tides in women's health. Throughout the decade more women put forward public discussions of their personal experiences with health generally and breast cancer specifically. As feminists argued, the personal was political, and women began to talk about their varied responses to breast cancer knowledge, detection, and treatment

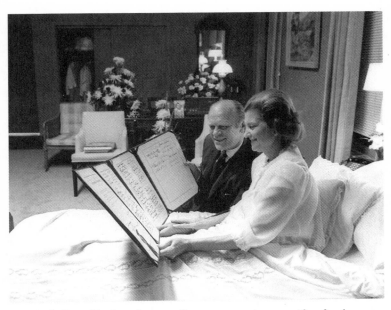

First Lady Betty Ford reads get-well messages and opens gifts after her mastectomy in 1974. (Courtesy of the Gerald R. Ford Library)

options.[11] Moreover, although the lump in Ford's breast was detected during a physical exam, it epitomized the value of early detection for the mass audiences who heard about her case. Few educators could have orchestrated a better plug for early detection of cancer, as Ford and her medical team continually reminded the public that early diagnosis increased rates of survival. In almost every media report, the value of early detection was reiterated. In addition, by 1974 the first clinical trials of mammography had been completed.[12] Due to their success, the ACS and National Cancer Institute expanded the study, opening it to the national population and recruiting women into the BCDDP. As women's awareness of breast cancer risk peaked in the wake of Ford's announcement, women jammed into mammography centers seeking access to screening technology. Betty Ford's breast cancer story encapsulates the persuasive influence of the personal medical narrative in the public discourse about women and cancer.

Mammography Reviewed

Throughout the 1960s the ACS, the NCI, the U.S. Public Health Service (USPHS), and others encouraged women to routinely examine their breasts, feeling breast tissue and searching for abnormal growths. Cancer awareness material advised women to conduct monthly breast self-examinations and to visit a physician with any abnormalities. Meanwhile, Philadelphia radiologist Dr. Jacob Gershon-Cohen was arguing that breast x-rays offered a more effective screening method for breast cancer. Screening women with x-ray, he contended, would allow patients to present at earlier stages of the disease and would improve survival rates.[13]

As early as 1937, Gershon-Cohen had invented a primitive form of mammography and published a paper indicating the diagnostic value of x-ray screening for breast cancer detection.[14] For the next two decades he adapted this x-ray technique, striving to make it more accurate, accessible, and safe. In 1956 Gershon-Cohen launched a five-year clinical trial at the Albert Einstein Medical Center in Philadelphia that screened over 1,000 asymptomatic women for breast cancer.[15]

In that same year Dr. Robert L. Egan, a radiologist from M. D. Anderson Hospital and Tumor Institute in Houston, Texas, had begun an independent mammography study. Also convinced that radiology could reveal earlier indications of breast cancer than palpation exams, Egan compared over 1,000 mammograms between 1956 and 1959. Using fine-grain industrial film, he studied suspicious masses and concluded that x-ray could yield at least two insights. First, mammography could determine if a growth were benign or malignant with greater than 90 percent accuracy. Second, mammograms revealed early malignancies that might still be undetectable by touch. Egan's studies prompted the USPHS to start clinical studies of mammography in twenty-four centers across the nation, focusing on its usefulness as a screening tool for breast cancer. The ACS and NCI would eventually add additional support for this research.[16]

Although Gershon-Cohen had shared his work with the scientific community in the 1930s, lay audiences did not learn about the potential of this screening tool until the 1960s, and widespread use of mammography did not occur until the 1970s. When the media did report on mammography in the early 1960s, it conveyed a positive view of x-ray as a sophisticated type of cancer screening. In a 1962 article, "New Weapons against Breast Cancer," published in *Ladies' Home Journal*, the journalist wrote that in the "hopefully near future," specialists might employ "special x-rays to detect it [breast cancer] even before it is discoverable to the touch."[17] After decades of rhetoric about the merits of early detection as the surest way to control and cure cancer, lay public audiences embraced notions of early screening devices.

The medical community was more divided in its response to mammography as a screening device. The loudest critics argued that the radiation exposure from the screening could itself be carcinogenic. Moreover, mammography yielded a high percentage of false positives, and the consequences of this error could include psychological trauma and, in the worst scenarios, unnecessary surgeries. Most of this criticism was pushed aside during the trials of the 1960s and the demonstration project of the early 1970s. In 1976, however, journalists exposed the heated debate within the medical community about the merits of mammography. As a result, the public became privy to the controversy over the cancer-causing implications of using radiation to screen women under the age of fifty and the outcomes of false positive diagnoses.[18]

Throughout the 1960s and early 1970s cancer awareness advocates tended to adhere to ACS recommendations. When the ACS celebrated mammography in 1973 as a major innovation for women and dedicated a large percentage of its research funds to this technology, female cancer advocates encouraged women to participate in the project. For the ACS and its supporters, the early challenges of mammography were common to those of any new medical technology. The ACS thus endorsed building new screening technology centers and training more technicians. The organization also focused on the task of proving the effectiveness of mammography and funding projects that would create better public access to the technology. (When the debate over the risks of mammography became public in 1976, the ACS found itself in the position of having to explain its enthusiastic support for this screening procedure.)

In the beginning, however, mammography was not portrayed as a technique for widespread use. Prior to the mid-1960s many public discussions of mammography presented the technology as limited in scope and applicability. Audiences of popular periodicals learned that x-ray screening was a select diagnostic tool. As *Reader's Digest* noted in 1962, if a manual breast examination conducted by a physician revealed a suspicious mass, "in all likelihood the physician will also want x-rays."[19] A 1963 article in the *Ladies' Home Journal* made the same point. As one patient related, "There was, Dr. B explained, a new diagnostic procedure which might be helpful in my case. Though it was just coming into use it had shown a high degree of accuracy in its results so far. In a case like mine, where the clinical findings were indicative, this could be the first, if not the added check needed to substantiate them. The technique was one of x-raying the breast."[20]

Within a few years, however, lay interest in the technology generated inquiries about its broader applicability. By May 1963, when *Good Housekeeping* published "The Better Way," journalists were suggesting that mammography could become a universal screening tool. This article described mammography as "a technique that is growing in use in detection of breast cancer" and intimated that x-ray provided earlier indications of cancer than manual self-examinations. The article included details about the history of x-ray and cancer and recent pilot studies on mammography screening, and it generated hope surrounding this new method of early detection. The voice of the ACS was expressed as cautiously optimistic: "Mammography, at present, does not *replace* a physical examination. However, many cancer experts believe it has great value as a diagnostic aid in conjunction with physical examination and the study of tissue from a tumor."[21]

The USPHS study and the trials of both Egan and Gershon-Cohen had offered positive reviews of mammography, which emphasized its reliability and accuracy. In 1963, inspired by the work of Gershon-Cohen and Egan, Philip Strax started the largest clinical trial yet of the mammogram. This trial included 62,000 women and compared breast cancer mortality among women who had mammograms and those who had not.[22] Funded by the NCI, Strax collaborated with statistician Sam Shapiro as a way to "prove" the effectiveness of mammography screening. Strax, Shapiro, and their colleagues concluded that mammography, as a screening tool for women over the age of fifty, could reduce mortality by as much as one-third. They advised routine mammography for breast cancer screening. By 1971, the results of this study had proved conclusive enough that Arthur Holleb of the ACS urged a large-scale demonstration project that would convince the public that this was an effective screening tool that should be implemented.[23]

In 1972 the ACS allocated $2 million for a demonstration project that would ultimately open twenty-seven centers in the United States and screen 270,000 asymptomatic women over the age of thirty-five for breast cancer. Called the Breast Cancer Detection Demonstration Project, the survey consisted of four parts: a medical interview, a physical breast exam by palpation, a mammogram, and a thermograph exam. The NCI, at the urging of director Dr. Frank Rauscher, agreed to cosponsor this project and allocated $5.4 million to support the testing centers.[24]

With such coordinated support, the trial began in 1973. Each of the over two dozen centers tested a minimum of 5,000 women during the first year and an additional 5,000 the second year. During the next year, the trial tracked the 10,000 participants.[25] The ACS reported, "Hopefully, as the ACS-NCI program develops over the next few years, we will discover how the benefits of careful clinical examination plus a medical history and diagnostic tests . . . can most practically and economically be brought to every woman at risk."[26] Historian Barron Lerner has argued that the ACS and proscreening advocates supported mammography because it fit within the cultural perception of cancer. "As we have seen," he writes, "early detection is consistent with American notions of risk aversion and individual responsibility for preventing disease."[27] Although science had provided evidence about the risk and fallacies of mammography, in the 1960s and early 1970s

American culture placed greater faith in technology that promised early detection.

At the same time that the public learned about the potential of mammography, advice literature urged women to continue conducting breast self-examinations (BSE). "Nothing replaces a careful physical examination," a *Redbook* journalist contended.[28] The ACS continued to encourage women to comply with cancer screening advice and BSE. Even in the heyday of technological advances for screening, much of the cancer awareness literature insisted that women maintain a vigilant watch for any cancer symptoms. As the *Redbook* author wrote, "For many years women have been bombarded by the media about the importance of self-examination of the breasts for early detection of cancer. The American Cancer Society has distributed many excellent leaflets on the value and methods of the examination. In spite of this, however, many women still do not carry out this necessary and often life-saving procedure."[29] Describing the BSE as "lifesaving," however, exaggerated the value of this method of cancer detection.

Like much of the mid-twentieth century literature that introduced clinical descriptions of breast self-examinations to large female audiences, this article repeated the steps for proper BSE. It described how women should methodically feel each quadrant of the breast while lying down. Although the author briefly noted recent innovative detection techniques, including mammography and thermography, like the ACS she urged readers to continue the breast self-examination. She concluded by reemphasizing her point and quelling any notions that mammography might replace personal vigilance: "In summary, careful, monthly self-detection of early breast cancer is probably one of the simplest, least expensive and most effective techniques we have available for early diagnosis and treatment."[30]

When Betty Ford was diagnosed with breast cancer in 1974, the BCDDP was already underway. Her diagnosis attracted national attention to the BCDDP, and soon after her diagnosis, women clamored to enroll in the project. Participation rates in the clinical study soared. At most centers more women applied for inclusion than could be accommodated. Ford's diagnosis, combined with the apparent success of mammography, transformed conventional wisdom about breast cancer and the significance of screening technology. Throughout 1975, mammography was publicly promoted and praised in popular American culture.

Several factors informed the evolution of early breast cancer screening in the 1970s. First, as Gershon-Cohen, Egan, Strax, and Shapiro demonstrated, many scientists believed that this technology could improve breast cancer detection. Ideally, earlier diagnosis would allow for treatment at the initial stages of the disease. Second, the largest funding agencies in the United States, including the NCI, USPHS, and the ACS, all had invested millions of research dollars into screening technology, and positive results from mammography trials would validate their spending and their emphasis on early detection. Screening technology reinforced the central motto of the ACS that early detection was a means to a cure.

In spite of these benefits, practical and medical concerns lingered. Scientists within the NCI questioned the safety of mammography. Mammography was expensive, and the clinical trials offered little in the way of cost-benefit analysis. Scientists also worried about its accuracy, especially the statistically significant false positives. Finally, theories varied about the age when mammography should begin, the frequency with which it should be applied, and the process that should be approved for a national health-care reform of this size and magnitude. Between 1975 and 1977 critics challenged the ACS and NCI on the front pages of American newspapers, and the ACS-NCI was forced to respond and reassure the public of the value of mammography.

A year after Betty Ford's diagnosis and the rush of women to enroll in the mammography project, the public learned about internal debates occurring within the ACS-NCI sponsored project. In 1975 John Bailer, the deputy associate director of the NCI and editor of the *Journal of the National Cancer Institute*, shared with the public his apprehension about the safety of mammography. Believing that x-rays could cause breast cancer, especially later in life for the young women being screened, he questioned the prudence of the BCDDP. Journalists picked up on this story and challenged the ACS and NCI to explain their support of the BCDDP. The public championed journalists' concerns about risk, safety measures, and informed consent.[31]

The ACS and NCI responded in several ways. Defending the project, they initiated further studies on the safety and effectiveness of mammography. The ACS hired Lester Breslow, dean of the University–California–Los Angeles School of Public Health, to review the data. In 1976 NCI director Frank Rauscher assembled 400 women who worked for the NCI to solicit their opinions on the matter. Unable to determine a clear consensus from the existent evidence, additional research was urged. In the meantime, the ACS-NCI adopted guidelines that included informing women of the risks involved due to radiation exposure and advising women under fifty to abandon routine screening.[32] As Daniel Greenberg commented in 1976, "The scientific and medical issues involved are complex and, in many instances, far from fully resolved, and decision making on the mammography question is not eased by the wide prevalence and public dread of the disease that the technique is intended to detect."[33] The public sought technologies that would allow for earlier detection, but the critics exposed the potential dangers hidden within the technologies.

For the next few years, cancer specialists, epidemiologists, statisticians, feminists, investigative journalists, and more pored over all material related to the BCDDP. "The BCDDP controversy," historian James Olson has written, "assumed the dimensions of a national scandal, with investigative reporters burrowing into NCI records in order to find a smoking gun of some kind, prima facie evidence that the American Cancer Society and the National Cancer Institute had jumped headlong into widespread mammography screening without pondering its possible consequences and perhaps even ignoring internal warnings."[34] The scandal of the mid-1970s sparked a wave of debate over mammography screening that would continue until the present day. Variables changed, including the introduction of mammography with low doses of radiation, yet the dispute over the promises and liabilities of cancer screening persisted.

Although these debates continued to surface throughout the 1980s and 1990s, mammography nevertheless dominated breast cancer detection because of its promise of detecting tumors earlier. Screening technology fueled a sense of optimism seeded by the nearly century-old devotion to early detection. Moreover, as the risks associated with radiation exposure lessened with technological improvements and more sophisticated knowledge, studies that emphasized the benefits of early screening gained more attention, and the ACS and others allowed women under the age of fifty to consider mammography screening at an earlier age for reasons such as "high risk."[35] As mammography centers opened across the country, medical insurance programs covered mammography, and ACS literature validated its claims, women participated in the technological transformation of cancer detection. Eventually, the federal government established standards for mammography to prevent fraudulent and abusive practices associated with the business of mammography.

Personal Stories and Public Responses

At the same time that medical professionals split over their opinions regarding mammography screening, surgeons debated the best treatment for breast cancer. Betty Ford's case again illustrated many of the tensions evident in breast cancer treatment in the early 1970s.

After announcing Ford's admittance to the hospital, White House press secretary Ron Nessen patiently fielded an array of questions about the procedure that would ensue. Many of the questions focused on the treatment options should Ford be diagnosed with breast cancer. By this time, 1974, physicians had conflicting opinions about the best course of treatment for breast cancer.[36] Moreover, former patients, most notably Rose Kushner, questioned the aggressiveness of traditional breast cancer treatment.

Diagnosed with breast cancer in 1973, Kushner criticized the procedural norms of breast cancer treatment. After refusing to consent to radical mastectomy at the same surgery as the biopsy (should it prove malignant), Kushner opted for a modified mastectomy. She visited eighteen surgeons who denied her request, before she located a surgeon who was willing to perform the more conservative surgery. With her personal experience as a case study, she demanded an explanation for the universality of the one-step mastectomy. Unable to find a satisfactory scientific explanation, she urged physicians to perform this procedure in two stages. Women could wake up from the biopsy, learn about the diagnosis, and then decide their course of treatment. In addition, Kushner exhorted women to become more effective patient advocates by learning about the disease, the definition of "stages" as indicated in diagnosis, and the various treatment options available to them.[37]

Kushner's work helped transform breast cancer treatment for women in the United States. Kushner provided a model whereby her personal exposé ignited political responses. She inspired others to share their stories of breast cancer and their frustrations with contemporary medical practice. Moreover, she worked to institutionalize medical changes for women so that all women could benefit from shifts that were occurring in individual medical settings. One of the most influential women's health advocates of the twentieth century, Kushner believed fervently that patients should have a voice in their diagnosis and treatment options.[38]

Recognizing the celebrity nature of Ford's case and the national attention leveled at every decision Ford made in 1974, Kushner repeatedly tried to reach Betty Ford to discuss the significance of her treatment choice. As a breast cancer survivor, author, and political activist, Kushner urged patients, in this case Betty Ford, to engage in critical evaluations of treatment decisions. She called the White House directly and desperately tried to have a conversation with the First Lady but without success. Instead, as Ron Nessen explained to the press, Ford would follow the standard procedure. If the biopsy indicated any malignancy, surgery would follow immediately.

Contentious medical debates, which had been ongoing since the late 1950s, highlighted the conflicting advice about the best course of treatment for women with breast cancer.[39] Although scientific evidence had begun to suggest that conservative mastectomy was as effective as radical surgery, the historical memory of William S. Halsted's influence and the public consciousness that linked cancer cure to excision created cultural resistance to the notion of conservative treatment. After conducting extensive research on breast cancer and reading multiple clinical studies of different treatment options, Kushner concluded that the one-step procedure failed to recognize the patient's rights and patient's voice. Moreover, multiple treatment options existed, including lumpectomy, standard mastectomy, and radical mastectomy; in general, women knew little about the differences between them. Like several medical practitioners who had adopted the theory that conservative treatment could be as effective as radical treatment, Kushner opposed the nondeliberate use of radical mastectomy. As historian Barron Lerner has described, Kushner launched a "one-woman crusade against the radical mastectomy and the one-step procedure." She recognized the cultural currency of Ford's decisions, and even after Nessen's announcement, she continued to call the White House with hopes that she could convince the First Lady to have a two-stage process.[40] Her efforts failed. Although she did not convince Ford to reconsider her treatment options, Kushner's quest to teach the public about breast cancer was effective, and by the mid-1970s Kushner was one of the leading critics of medical protocol on women's health.[41]

The public learned about Ford's cancer diagnosis and subsequent treatment almost immediately. After her mastectomy, her doctors— Dr. William Lukash, the White House physician; Dr. William Fouty, chairman of surgery at the National Naval Medical Center; and Dr. J. Richard Thistlethwaite, a professor of surgery at George Washington University—shared the results of Ford's operation at a press conference. Lukash started the conference, "I am sorry to have to report today that the nodule in Mrs. Ford's breast was found to be malignant and as a result, surgical removal of the breast was required." He quickly added, "I am optimistic that the overall prognosis will be excellent." Fouty, a surgeon who believed in aggressive treatment, then described that he had completed a standard radical mastectomy on the First Lady. Relaying the information in a factual tone, he explained that the tumor was "approximately two centimeters in size." The operation removed Ford's pectoral muscles and lasted over two hours; Ford had awakened to learn of her diagnosis.[42]

Reporters immediately zeroed in on Ford's treatment options. Breast cancer survivors such as Kushner, who had publicly expressed their dissatisfaction with the one-step mastectomy, had directed media attention to this topic and to the controversy surrounding treatment options.[43] As one reporter asked:

> Q: Did Mrs. Ford have any choice? Did she have any
>   say before as to what would happen?
> Dr. Lukash: She was in discussion with us when we
>   all met with the President at the White House, and
>   she was in full agreement.
> Q: And she gave the green light for any—
> Dr. Lukash: Yes, sir.
> Q: She was told of the different procedures that were
>   possible and was she told some doctors believe that
>   simple mastectomy might be enough?
> Dr. Lukash: Yes.

Although Ford's decision to have a one-step procedure disappointed many, the media coverage introduced this discussion of treatment options to a large population. By focusing on the debates surrounding the one- and two-step mastectomy and by exposing the medical controversy about necessary treatment, the media coverage pushed discussions of breast cancer in new directions that were less exclusively grounded in early detection rhetoric.[44]

Ford's choices were particularly disappointing to feminist health activists who had been challenging the basis of medical authority for several years. For example, women from the Buffalo Women's Self-Help Clinic wrote to Ford, "We question the rapidity of the medical diagnosis in your case, and the absence of any time for you to evaluate, obtain additional medical advice or consider alternatives to radical mastectomy."[45] Throughout the late 1960s and early 1970s, women organized themselves in the name of women's rights, gender equality, and feminism. Activists concerned about women's health insisted that women needed to employ their agency in order to influence health-care decisions that affected their bodies. The enormous success of the feminist health manual *Our Bodies, Ourselves*, a handbook written by and for women, offered one indication that many women shared a desire to learn more about health issues.[46] For many who were invested in breast cancer activism in the early 1970s, radical surgery was a misogynist medical practice that should be abandoned in favor of more conservative surgery.

Additional questions at the press conference about Ford's surgery embodied various perceptions of breast cancer in contemporary American culture. For instance, one reporter implied that a radical operation must have meant that the cancer had been widespread. When the reporter asked the doctor about it, Fouty answered, diplomatically, "There are different types of mastectomy. The standard procedure, and accepted procedure, for carcinoma of the breast of this type would be removal of the breast with the muscle and lymphoid tissue."[47] With Ford's diagnosis and the media coverage that surrounded it, controversies about mastectomy became embedded in public discussions of breast cancer, and the public cast a newly critical lens toward previously accepted medical standards.

For days, the media prioritized Ford's diagnosis and treatment as a "top story." NBC evening news anchor Tom Brokaw and correspondent John Cochran reported the details of the operation. In addition to presenting medical descriptions to millions of television viewers, some commentators began a discussion of Ford's decision to make her personal health concerns public information. ABC commentator Harry Reasoner, analyzing the value of an open and public discussion of cancer, concluded, "The case of Betty Ford shows even more dramatically how far we have come because we are not only talking about cancer, we are talking about a breast, and that used to be a word only a little less taboo than cancer."[48]

To be sure, although Reasoner perceived breasts and cancer as taboo subjects, both had found their way into newsprint, radio shows, women's clubs, popular periodicals, and the like for decades. Yet, the celebrity status of the First Lady directed an unprecedented amount of media attention to one case of breast cancer. Moreover, although the media discussion was based on an individual encounter with cancer, much of the coverage addressed general issues of women's risk, treatment, detection, and more—cultivating a sense of community among women who shared vulnerability to this dreaded disease. The conversations that emerged, between Ford's press team and reporters, between Rose Kushner and public audiences, among women in health collectives, all indicated that the personal could be political. Cancer awareness had been growing throughout the twentieth century, but this publicity was unexpected, unplanned, and hugely beneficial to all concerned about expanding the dialogue about women's health and the messages of early detection. Reasoner's comments, like those of many media commentators in 1974, reflected his unfamiliarity with earlier efforts to teach women about breast and uterine cancers. Although he perpetuated the myth that no one discussed female cancers publicly before the 1970s, he also created a new venue where cancer awareness issues could reach a far larger audience—television.

Ford received telegrams of condolence, prayer, and support from across the globe. Politicians expressed their sympathy, and all one hundred senators signed a formal greeting that wished Betty Ford luck and a speedy recovery.[49] Ford's diagnosis also prompted approximately 55,000 people to write letters to the First Lady, expressing both concern and gratitude. The letters Ford received can be placed into two broad categories. Some people wrote to commend her courage and express appreciation for her open discussion of breast cancer. Others, who were breast cancer survivors, shared their personal experiences with Ford and offered her advice about postoperative care. This latter set of letters provides a unique insight into how individual women identified themselves as "breast cancer survivors."

Very few people criticized Ford's decision to make her disease public. A sample of the letters written to Ford, housed at the Ford

Library, records overwhelming public support for her decision.[50] "I want you to know how much I admire you and the President. You for your strength and courage during the illness, which to my great sadness fell upon you," one woman wrote.[51] Another woman wrote, "And, then to have had that operation—you look terrific and beautiful after going through so very much and you've held your head high. Thank God you are all right! My prayers were for you, and still are. . . . Thank you, Betty, for listening to me."[52] Others applauded Ford for the lives she saved. "My reason for writing you," one confided, "is to let you know that you actually saved my mother's life."[53] Another woman wrote that she was "terribly sorry about your illness last year. It was a high price to pay but you can take credit, and I hope comfort, in the fact that thousands of women in the nation are having examinations and not letting similar conditions occur without discovery in time for treatment."[54] Many young Americans wrote her also. A sixteen-year-old girl wrote, "I admire your courage in facing surgery the way you did and in making it public. You have probably saved more lives than you will ever realize."[55] A seventh-grade student informed the First Lady, "I thought you would be interested to know that I chose as my project 'Breast Cancer' since I had read in the newspapers and heard on the radio and T.V. news casts about your recent surgery."[56] Other typical letters included inquiries about Ford's treatment, praise for her courage, and concern for her health.

Ford inspired a variety of women to write. Several self-identified black women used the opportunity to share their concerns with the First Lady. "I am a black woman," wrote one, who shared her best wishes with Ford as she told her about personal health concerns, including a spinal problem.[57] Another woman explained that Ford's diagnosis had inspired her and influenced her thesis on race and cancer, "Incidences of Breast Cancer and the Psychological Effects in Black Women."[58] Ford's popularity and the publicity given to this diagnosis nurtured a sense of shared experiences among women concerned about cancer in particular and health more generally.

The Ford Library has estimated that women who identified themselves as breast cancer survivors wrote approximately 10 percent of the letters sent to Ford.[59] Many women poured out their hearts in these letters, relating their intimate reactions to breast cancer and chronicling their personal experiences with the disease. "Dear Mrs. Ford, If this will help I want you to know that I had a radical mastectomy in July 17 years [ago] and have had no recurrence." After explaining many facets of her experience, she continued, "Sorry to go into so much detail but I feel sure you will get along as well as I have as the circumstances seem so similar, and I wish to assure you. We discovered it in time."[60] Another woman wrote, "I hope you won't think me presumptuous in referring to your recent operation. You see, Shirley Temple Black and I invite you to join the Club, there are many members as you know. I had the same operation in June 1960. As an entertainer and being in public life, I must confess it was a traumatic experience at the time, however it was absolutely necessary and I shall be forever grateful for the happy life I have been living ever since. I went back to work (making a TV series with my husband) six weeks after the operation. It was great therapy."[61]

This writer's reference to the "club" reflects a growing sense of community among breast cancer survivors. Although notions of identity as cancer survivors first became evident in a small and general way in the late 1930s with the Cured Cancer Club, and Terese Lasser's creation of Reach to Recovery in 1954 had first offered a formal support network to breast cancer survivors, others found support in an imagined community that now included celebrity survivor Betty Ford. Friends and family and others provided additional informal support networks.

One aspect of the survivor community included a dialogue about post-treatment concerns, most notably advice about dealing with the effects of mastectomy. Several survivors who wrote to Ford shared advice about breast prosthesis. For example, one letter read, "Fifteen yrs ago I had a radical mastectomy—(at age 61) fitted with a prosthesis (false breast) having fluid—which in a short time deflated—and I hurried to make one—(of foam rubber-soft cloth with cotton between the layers)—placing this in the pocket sewn to the under side of the BRA—by sewing machine on 3 sides and snaps on the top—for easy removal of the said breast) that the bra may be laundered."[62]

Another wrote to Ford to impart knowledge that she had gained through a friend. As she explained, "A friend who had a mastectomy 18 years ago has tried every kind of prosthesis made. She says the only satisfactory one is the silicone one by Airway Surgical Co., Cincinnati. It is very good. If you don't like it next to your skin, put it in the case from the Reach to Recovery people. They will be happy to get you more of them."[63] Still others wanted to share their custom-designed prostheses with Ford. Dolores Smith assured Ford that the results of the mastectomy could be addressed. A "totally new concept that not only corrects the physical, but . . . the psychological aspects of this type of surgery," could be found through Smith's "Surgical Mastectomy Bra Design #1." This bra held a prosthetic breast and thereby restored a woman's "female form" after surgery. Smith believed a prosthetic breast would allow Ford to look and feel "normal" after her breast amputation. As she concluded, "Looking physically the same after operation softens the traumatic deep shock of radical surgery."[64] Smith's concern for "restoring" Ford's female figure was hardly unique. Reach to Recovery had also sent Ford its literature and emphasized similar points about the importance of a good prosthetic breast.

Several women even requested permission to visit Ford. One woman wrote to President Ford, "I would very much like to visit your wife at Bethesda Naval Hospital. Having had a radical mastectomy in 1970 at Quantico Naval Hospital, I would appreciate the opportunity to help reassure her on the probability of complete recovery and ability to return to her usual activities."[65] Finally, women wrote to offer Ford empathy. One woman explained, "Like millions of other people, my sincere thoughts are with you. You and I now have two things in common. We both serve on the Board of Governors of the Capitol Hill Club, with you as our first Vice President, and we both have experienced mastectomy. When my radical mastectomy was performed in 1952 it was determined terminal, with six months to live. They administered maximum radiation, and here I am writing you, 22 years later. At the time of my surgery I knew no one who had undergone the same experience."[66] Convinced that camaraderie existed because of their shared experiences, women like these offered their time and stories to the First Lady.

For many women, Betty Ford served as an inspiration. For others, she acted as a spokesperson for the women's health movement by directing more attention to female cancers. Clearly, her diagnosis introduced the subject of breast cancer to co-ed audiences, removing it from the female spaces it had occupied for many decades. Yet her diagnosis resonated in particular with women. As these letters clearly suggest, women felt a connection to the First Lady. By merely discussing her breast cancer diagnosis with mass audiences, she reminded Americans that women's health was a national concern. As the First Lady, Ford opened the doors for inquiry about the status of mammography screening, the availability of diagnostic tools for all women, and the need for continued attention to women's health.

Three weeks after Ford's diagnosis, Happy Rockefeller announced her diagnosis for breast cancer, which fueled further publicity for the disease. Happy Rockefeller's diagnosis stunned much of the nation. It followed Ford's case so closely that any sense that Ford was an anomaly quickly disappeared. Instead, Rockefeller's diagnosis seemed to convince women of the high risk that breast cancer posed.

Five weeks later, the public consciousness about breast cancer was further heightened when Rockefeller returned to the hospital for a second mastectomy, this time an excision of her right breast. As her husband, Governor Rockfeller, explained at the press conference (which Happy Rockefeller opted to skip), a routine biopsy of her right breast had been performed during her initial surgery. It revealed "a pinhead of malignant cells."[67] Although the cells appeared "dormant," Happy Rockefeller complied with medical advice that suggested "the best thing, the safest thing, the surest thing was to have a second operation."[68] Many people throughout the United States wrote letters of support to Happy Rockefeller. As she recalled, "I was completely unprepared for the thoughtfulness of strangers. I received an astonishing flood of letters from people I'd never met—thousands upon thousands of letters wishing me well."[69] Ford's and Rockefeller's public discussions of breast cancer not only evoked sympathetic responses but served to direct increased attention to the importance of early breast cancer detection and prompt treatment.

Breast Cancer Diagnoses and Treatment Options

In 1954 Dr. Edward J. McCormick, American Medical Association president, admonished surgeons: "Simple mastectomy [the removal of the breast without simultaneously removing adjacent lymph glands] is to be condemned. Complete excision of the breast and axillary contents is absolutely necessary if cure is expected."[70] Some physicians took these ideas a step further, performing super-radical mastectomies that left women disfigured. The effects were multifaceted. As physician and historian Barron Lerner has written, "In addition to the extensive tissue loss that accompanied a standard radical mastectomy, women undergoing the procedure were left with a permanent defect in the rib cage that created a marked concavity in the center of their chests."[71] At the same time that remarkable innovations in science and technology after World War II were convincing many that cancer could be cured, age-old conventional wisdom about treatment persisted. Many surgeons still considered radical surgery the key to curing cancer.

In Europe, however, physicians had been opting for more conservative surgery for years, and by the end of the 1940s several physicians had published data that proved that radical and conservative surgeries yielded similar outcomes. Geoffrey Keynes of London concluded as early as 1924 that the Halsted radical surgery was no more effective than modified mastectomies. Convinced that radiation could complement conservative surgery and produce better survival rates, Keynes urged surgeons to abandon the radical operation in the later 1940s. Robert McWhirter of Edinburgh shared Keynes's philosophy and published data in 1949 that demonstrated the effectiveness of conservative surgery. Likewise, David Patey and W. H. Dyson of Middlesex published evidence that indicated extensive surgeries generated no additional benefits for the patients. Although these physicians attracted some converts, in the United States many surgeons remained wedded to radical surgery, still convinced that breast cancer was a local growth and extensive removal of the surrounding area secured the best odds for recovery.[72]

In 1970, therefore, most American physicians continued to treat breast cancer with a radical mastectomy; Ford's case was no anomaly.[73] This process typically involved the removal of the breast, the underlying muscles of the chest wall, all the glands in the armpit, and all other glands underneath the muscles in the chest wall. The radical mastectomy took between two and four hours, included a recovery period of several days, produced significant deformity in the chest, and led to cases of lymphedema (swelling of the arm) in approximately 20 percent of women. The cure rate after treatment with radical mastectomy, which was based on a five-year survival rate, hovered around 70 percent.

The majority of American surgeons, convinced that breast cancer needed to be treated as immediately and aggressively as possible, dismissed critics of the radical mastectomy, reproaching them for failing to treat women with the best standard of care. Several critics faced hostility from professional audiences. In the United States George (Barney) Crile of the Cleveland Clinic and Bernard Fisher of the University of Pittsburgh nevertheless challenged the merits of radical operations. In spite of their vocal criticism, it took decades to transform the practical treatment of cancer.[74]

Beginning in 1970, critics of radical surgery gained a broader audience. One determining factor in this trend was women's response to the medical debate. Unable to convert surgeons, many critics of radical mastectomy turned to lay female audiences to share their theories and data. At the urging of feminists, Dr. Oliver Cope, a surgeon who had been performing modified surgeries since the 1950s, published his findings in *Radcliffe Quarterly* so that lay female audiences could learn about the voracious debate within medical circles.

Critics continued to probe medical audiences as well. At the annual meeting of the American College of Surgeons in the fall of 1970, Barney Crile presented a paper that favored conservative breast cancer surgery. After more than a decade of treating breast cancer patients with lumpectomy and radiation, and achieving survival statistics that equaled Halsted's, Crile challenged the merits of radical mastectomy. Moreover, he stressed that, among its many benefits, conservative surgery proved much less invasive and traumatizing to patients. Crile's procedure involved the simple removal of the cancerous lump, took about ten minutes, produced minor scarring, and allowed the patient to return home in two days. In addition to sharing his medical results, Crile reproached physicians for marginalizing women's voices. Fully aware that many feminists supported his studies, and also aware that his presentation would draw harsh criticism from traditionalists in medical circles, Crile openly welcomed patients to participate in this dialogue.[75]

Shortly after the conference, in April 1971, *McCall's* published an article by Dr. William Nolen, a surgeon who had followed Crile's advice by adopting conservative breast cancer surgery. Nolen bluntly stated, "I think the time has come when women should have something to say about what operation she wants . . . a lumpectomy, or simple, radical, or bilateral mastectomy." In order to support this medical opinion, Nolen shared one of his personal experiences with a breast cancer patient. During a manual exam of this patient, he discovered that, "deep in her left breast, above and to the outside of the nipple, there was a hard lump about the size of a marble." After he told the patient what he had found, he encouraged her to feel the lump herself, and then the physician and patient discussed the situation. He explained that the breast lump was probably not malignant but that biopsy offered the only definitive diagnosis. If the biopsy indicated cancer, treatment would be immediate and include removal of her breast. He advised his patient to think about it, discuss it with her family, and return for another visit.[76]

The patient returned for a biopsy, and Nolen learned the tumor was malignant. As he described the next step:

So, proceeding almost automatically, I did the operation we surgeons have been doing for breast cancer for
the last fifty years—the so-called radical mastectomy.
I removed Jean's entire left breast, the underlying
muscles on her chest wall, and all the small bean-
shaped glands—the lymph glands—in her left armpit.
As a result of this surgery, Jean was in the hospital for
ten days, has the obvious cosmetic deformity that goes
with the loss of one breast, and has a left arm that is
about 20 percent thicker than her right. And yet in all
the tissue I removed there wasn't one cancer cell: simple
removal of the lump would have done as much to cure
Jean as my radical mastectomy.[77]

By the time Nolen wrote this article, he regretted that choice of treatment. "In the future," he declared, "my patients with breast cancer, if
they wish, are going to join me in making the decision."[78]

Through this narrative of regret, Nolen addressed the controversy
of breast cancer surgery and admitted that no single "best" option existed. Surgeons throughout the country might perform any number
of operations, ranging from a superradical mastectomy to a lumpectomy. The three categories of operation most frequently referred to in
popular discourse were radical mastectomy, simple mastectomy, and
lumpectomy. Nolen informed his readers that anyone making treatment decisions should consider many factors, including a patient's
age, the location of cancer, and the patient's family history. Moreover, he openly recognized the uncertainty of any cancer diagnosis
and experience. As an example, he explained that he had treated a
woman with advanced breast cancer and a family history of the disease, expecting the cancer to metastasize within six months. Instead,
ten years later, the patient was alive and well, "which shows, hap-
pily, how wrong I—or any other surgeon—can be about cancer of the
breast."[79] The medical controversies of the 1970s had created a forum
that exposed the uncertainties of science and medicine and offered a
sophisticated discussion of treatment options.

In 1973 the ACS explicitly joined this discussion with its production of a film called *Breast Cancer: Where We Are*. The film traced changes in public awareness of breast cancer through the previous six decades, emphasizing the importance of breast self-examination. Featuring female models, journalists, and others who openly confessed concerns about breast cancer, the film captured a variety of women who wanted to know more about breast cancer than simple messages of early detection.[80]

Very early in the film, the camera zooms in on John Mack Carter, the editor of *Ladies' Home Journal*. Recognizing the magazine's historical commitment to advancing cancer awareness since 1913, Carter suggests, "In spite of effort, an aura of mystery shrouds the disease and an aura of mystery shrouds the female form. People haven't wanted to talk about the one or reveal the other." By referencing a history of neglect, the editor pointed to the need for contemporary concern and elicited the audience to engage in more open discussion of the female body and cancer. In point of fact, women had been working to demystify cancer for decades, but education campaigns had not talked about cancer in the ways that the public in the 1970s wanted. More significant, prior to the 1970s female-centered cancer awareness efforts cooperated with the medical profession and even advanced its professional project. The critical edge of the 1970s discussion was revolutionary. Carter's reference to 1913 recalls the legacy of cancer awareness efforts that targeted women, but it also suggests why these efforts had failed to attract the audiences now sought by the 1970s programs. Specifically, he wanted to broaden the discussion of women, cancer, and illness so that women could understand the tension in contemporary medical debates better.

The film then shifts its focus to a second magazine contributor, Helen Gurley Brown. Brown of *Cosmopolitan* explains, "I think women are terrified about it [breast cancer]." *Cosmopolitan* decided to publish articles that would teach its predominantly female readers how to perform BSE and to print narratives about patients' experiences. The magazine had experienced the greatest success with this effort when it printed a story about a woman who had undergone a double mastectomy. In this narrative the patient addressed public concerns about losing a breast, changes in the body, and worries about intimacy and sexuality after mastectomy.

Returning to public personalities, the narrator of the film interviews nationally syndicated advice columnist Ann Landers, who by the early 1970s was encouraging her readers to conduct breast self-examinations. After first addressing this topic in her column, 250,000 readers wrote a response to Landers. For decades, women involved in cancer awareness had created forums for public discussions of cancer. Women's magazines published stories about BSE, and the BSE film was viewed by hundreds of thousands of women. Yet, Landers's forum touched a broader audience than these and reflected the importance of shifts in cancer discussions in the 1970s. Many women embraced the public campaigns about contemporary breast cancer and considered the attention directed to cancer as remarkably different than that of the past.

Breast Cancer: Where We Are then shifts its attention to medical topics. It describes the breast self-examination and Pap smear as screening tools that allow women to detect cancer at its earliest stage. The narrator notes the emergence of new diagnostic techniques for breast cancer, including mammography, thermography, and xerography, but also stressed the importance of all women continuing to conduct the breast self-examination monthly.[81]

The ACS and other cancer educators assured women that the BSE was simple and quick. One BSE promotion encouraged women to conduct breast self-examinations while showering. Embedded within the film was a 1973 television commercial that featured a woman showering behind foggy glass. The narrator states:

> If you are a woman what you are about to see might
> save your life. Once a month, just once a month, while
> you are taking a shower and you have a few moments,
> before you dry or spray or do any of those little things
> to pamper yourself—do something to take care of your-
> self. Examine your breasts. That's where it begins. It's

a nothing examination really. It's uncomplicated, it doesn't hurt, and only takes about two minutes. If you don't know how, ask your doctor to show you, or ask us, the ACS. We'll send you a simple little leaflet that shows you. . . . Two minutes of your life, once a month, is very cheap insurance. Don't you think? Don't be afraid. It's what you don't know that can hurt you. Please call.

The rising endorsement of the BSE and the variety of public personas that supported its promotion validated the merits of this screening tactic. Yet, the rhetoric surrounding these health messages for women continued to patronize female audiences. Often relying on gendered images of dependency, the messages frequently sounded like advice to children. As one example, the aforementioned advertisement deemed this procedure lifesaving and told women it was "uncomplicated" and "didn't hurt," as if women would refuse to conduct the exam if it were not simple.

Although the film reflected the rising impulse of the feminist movement that insisted that women have more control of their bodies and health care, stereotypical norms pervaded these messages. Screening technology was celebrated, and failures that resulted from it were often linked to women's unwillingness to comply with screening guidelines. In the final scenes of the film, as in previous dramas produced by the ACS, the film traces one patient's experience with a medical exam. In a significant shift from earlier cancer awareness films, the woman concerned about cancer visits a female physician. This doctor appears nurturing and caring, attributes stereotypically described as feminine. For instance, she holds the patient's hand and maintains eye contact with the patient while explaining the exam. Whereas many earlier films that featured male physicians reinforced the different positions of the patient and physician, this film focused more on the personal relationship between the doctor and patient and less on the actual exam.[82]

The film ends on an optimistic note. It emphasizes that researchers were constantly improving detection methods. It also includes a brief discussion of the physical and emotional effects of treatment. For example, it praises the work of Reach to Recovery: "We can't over-estimate what visits mean to the patient." As indicated in the opening scene, the film includes some racial diversity throughout, although it still seems dominated by middle-class women. In one of the closing scenes, six patients, two of whom are black, discuss their diagnosis and treatment.

The shifts evident in this 1973 film are remarkable for several reasons. First, it placed women at the center. It portrayed a female medical authority and featured influential women who promised to publicize the BSE. However, the film also echoed early cancer aware-ness campaigns by praising the BSE and reinforcing cultural notions of blame by insisting that women who performed BSE would be safe. It reflected a community of women talking to one another without challenging any medical paradigms. Finally, it valorized the medi-cal profession by claiming that its research would advance screening technology in the near future.

The Women's Health Movement of the Late 1960s and Early 1970s

In the late 1960s women organized and challenged the patri-archal structure of American society. As feminists critiqued gender inequalities apparent throughout society, women shared common experiences with one another and recognized similar frustrations with access to power. Historian Sarah Evans has observed, "The cen-tral organizing tool of the women's liberation movement, the small consciousness-raising group, proved an effective mechanism for movement building."[83]

Soon after the women's liberation movement started in the late 1960s, many feminists discussed concerns about their health. As one woman remembered, "We had all experienced similar feelings of frustrations and anger toward specific doctors and the medical gaze in general, and initially we wanted to do something about those doctors who were condescending, paternalistic, judgmental, and non-informative."[84] Other scholars have noted, "The medicalization of so many aspects of the female life cycle (pregnancy, menopause, etc.), not to mention the use of medical arguments to justify the exclusion of women from certain occupations, literally forced feminists to make health a central arena for struggle."[85]

Much of the early concern for women's health, addressed at the 1967 meeting of the National Organization of Women, focused on debates about women's access to reproductive rights. "The abortion struggle provided the initial impetus for a broader women's health movement by creating widespread awareness of how medical and legal systems obstruct women's right to control their own fertility," Sheryl Burt Ruzek has written.[86] By 1971, efforts to inform women about their health included much broader matters. For example, in a Los Angeles bookstore in 1971, Carol Downer inserted a speculum into her vagina and allowed others to learn about the cervix by observing hers. As Ruzek describes it, "self-help gynecology" allowed women to "reclaim parts of themselves controlled by male professionals."[87] As self-help gynecology spread to different regions of the country, it also taught women to examine their breasts for cancer. Some discussion emerged about how women might perform their own Pap smears, but most vaginal smears remained confined to physicians' offices and clinics.[88] Although cancer was not a central concern during the initial years of the women's health movement, the movement's resolve to familiarize women with their bodies reinforced the emphasis that cancer awareness advocates placed on early detection. With its political angle, however, the women's health movement also recast the discussion on the politics of the body and the marginalization of women's health in the U.S. health-care system.

As one indication of the long-term impact of this transitional moment, several informal women's health organizations that emerged in the late 1960s and early 1970s became institutionalized over time. For example, beginning in 1969, several women in the northeastern United States gathered to discuss health and women's bodies. Dubbing themselves the "doctor's group," these women shared their experiential knowledge of health and soon augmented this information with research on medical subjects. To learn more, every member of the collective researched and wrote papers on different topics. Ultimately, these papers turned into a course, "Women and Their Bodies," and by 1971 this course became the popular book, *Our Bodies, Our Selves: A Course by and for Women*, authored by the Boston Women's Health Collective and published by the New England Free Press. The book reflected the authors' concerns about the current medical system, which tended to treat women as passive patients. It discussed a myriad of medical issues that defined women's lives, including female anatomy, sexuality, and reproduction. As the authors explained, "We talked about our own experiences and we shared our own knowledge. We went to books and to medically trained people for more information. We decided on the topics collectively."[89] To the authors' delight and dismay, women across the country read the booklet, told other women about it, and bought copies of it. By 1973, the collective offered Simon and Schuster publication rights because the demand had exceeded the capabilities of the original press. By then, it had already been through eleven printings by the small New England press, and over 225,000 copies had been sold.[90]

In 1971 the first edition of *Our Bodies, Our Selves* included no information on cancer. In twelve sections that covered topics such as venereal disease, birth control, abortion, pregnancy, and medical institutions, the book offered its initial evaluation of major women's health concerns. The authors realized the limits of this edition and included a preface in reprints that read, "The first printing sold out so fast we haven't had time to revise the printed course. We are working on revisions that we hope will be ready for the 3rd printing." They added, "We want to expand the existing chapters to include more on monogamy, homosexuality, women's diseases and hysterectomies."[91]

In 1973 the collective published a revised version of the course book, *Our Bodies, Ourselves: A Book by and for Women*. This edition included four pages of information on breast and cervical cancer within the chapter, "Women and Health Care." The section opened, "The thought of any kind of cancer is terrifying to most of us. As women we are particularly concerned with cancer of the breasts or reproductive organs. If we get one of these cancers, not only do we have to face our own mortality, but even when we recover, the treatment may mean the loss of a part of us that has played an important role in out definition of ourselves."[92] Much of the information on breast and cervical cancer in the book echoed the rhetoric of the ACS. It encouraged regular breast self-examinations and Pap smears and admonished women who delayed medical consultation, labeling this action "foolish." It listed the standard treatment options for cancer as well. However, unlike the ACS, this early edition of *Our Bodies, Ourselves* also facilitated a discussion of cancer care that empowered patients by encouraging them to question standard treatment and to contribute to their diagnostic decisions. It reminded readers that the doctor needed their permission before performing any treatment. Further, it suggested that lumpectomy and simple mastectomy might be as effective as a radical operation. It concluded, "The most important thing to remember is that breast cancer is still not very well understood, that probably no one treatment is clearly the best one, and that your feelings about losing a breast or receiving radiation or taking general anesthesia are all important considerations in making any decision."[93]

The 1976 "revised and expanded" edition offered twice as many pages of information on breast and cervical cancers within a chapter section titled "Common Medical and Health Problems—Traditional and Alternative Treatments." It included an extended discussion of cancer causes and risk factors and urged women to perform the breast self-examination regularly. Unlike many popular discussion of breast cancer, however, it identified the culpability of medical professionals. Women should demand a breast examination from doctors, authors advocated, and ask physicians to demonstrate proper techniques for BSE. As the authors said, "Your health is not in your doctor's hands, it is in yours."[94] *Our Bodies* described a range of breast abnormalities, and similar to most cancer literature, it reminded women that the vast majority of lumps in the breast were not cancerous. It also re-

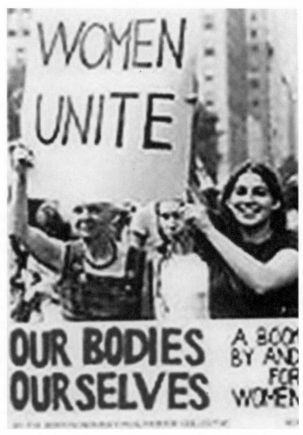

Front cover of the 1973 edition of the feminist health manual, *Our Bodies, Ourselves*. (Courtesy of the Schlesinger Library, Radcliffe Institute for Advanced Study, Cambridge, Mass.)

minded women to have annual Pap smears and detailed the meaning of the "class" in cervical cancer diagnosis, a term used to indicate the stage of the cancer.

The 1976 edition also presented emerging medical studies that challenged the necessity of radical mastectomies, and convinced by these findings, the authors suggested that women consider a simple mastectomy. "DO NOT ALLOW YOURSELF TO BE STAMPEDED INTO SUR-GERY," they insisted.[95] At the very least, the authors hoped women would insist on a two-stage mastectomy to allow time for consideration of all treatment options. Finally, the 1976 *Our Bodies, Ourselves* invited women to share their experiences with other women, use the support network provided by Reach to Recovery, and learn about the procedures being performed.[96]

The women's health movement critiqued a medical system that placed men in positions of power. It challenged the expertise of professional medicine and the assumption that laypersons, especially women, could not learn the scientific and technical aspects of health, bodies, and treatment. It argued that the medical system depended on models of illness versus wellness, tended to objectify women, and administered health care through a capitalist model that prioritized profits. It urged women to learn as much as possible about their own bodies, challenge traditional treatment, and demand a voice in their health care. As *Our Bodies, Ourselves* spelled out in its 1973 preface, "For us, body education is core education. Our bodies are the physical bases from which we move out into the world; ignorance, uncertainty—even, at worst, shame—about our physical selves create in us an alienation from ourselves that keeps us from being the whole people that we could be."[97] In the next several decades, women with such feminist sensibilities contributed to debates on mammography, vaginal smears, cancer, funding and research, patient access to care, and much more.

The mammography debates that began in the 1960s continued in subsequent decades and still exist today. As a 2002 newspaper article read, "If you are confused about what the best science says about the value of mammograms for women at normal risk for breast cancer, you are in excellent company."[98] Indicative of the enormous changes that took place in the final decades of the twentieth century, cancer awareness information became informed by medical and scientific theory. The public, women's health advocates in particular, consumed this information and responded to it collectively. When a

2002 Danish study cast doubt on mammography, readers responded from an informed standpoint and activist consciousness that demanded explanation and information. The public learned details that in earlier decades may have remained relegated to the pages of medical journals. As Jane Brody explained, "It has been said that the only certainties in life are death and taxes. And so, it appears, we are likely to have to ensure continued declarations of uncertainty about the health-saving and lifesaving benefits of screening mammography, which has been mired in controversy for decades."[99] Women who wanted comprehensive breast cancer information in the mid-1970s organized, creating influential advocacy groups in the 1980s that ensured that medical debates related to their bodies and health would merit national attention and solicit their responses.[100]

In spite of the renewed discussion of breast cancer, many other female cancers remained marginalized. For instance, the public learned little about ovarian cancer, and emerging screening techniques failed in early diagnosis. A gynecology professor described the delay in understanding ovarian cancer as reprehensible at a Chicago medical convention in 1964, explaining that as many as 50 percent of ovarian cancers were not discovered until it was too late to operate. Dr. Albert Lorincz advocated prompt removal of all ovarian cysts because of the difficulty of determining malignant cysts and the likelihood that a malignant cyst might lead to death.[101] Medical controversy aside, one reason that activists may have directed little attention to ovarian cancer is that early detection rhetoric had little resonance for this cancer.

The feminist health movement introduced strategies to change all aspects of women's health. It encouraged women to organize, meet, and discuss concerns about their bodies. Activists engaged in legislative issues, public policy, and judicial changes that would benefit them. Feminists called for greater evaluations of the merits of simple and radical mastectomy and hysterectomy. Finally, the women's health movement created an environment that allowed for an open discussion of women's bodies and health, thereby dismantling the two perceptions that may have hindered a wider public discussion of women's cancers before 1970—the hesitancy to discuss breasts and vaginas and lingering reluctance to discuss cancer publicly. As Betty Ford's 1974 reaction to her breast cancer diagnosis demonstrated, the women's health movement indeed redefined the parameters of the public recognition of women's bodies and women's health.

For women devoted to cancer education, the 1970s marked a divisive, challenging, and exciting moment. Within this context of political activism, the early educational campaigns based on a message of early detection seemed both simple and naive. Cancer involved much more than recognition of early symptoms. Women sought answers to complex questions about this disease and public health concerns. How does one determine the best treatment option? Why are more black women dying from breast cancer even though more white women are diagnosed with it? How do women without health insurance receive cancer screening? As questions about access to mammography and vaginal smears emerged, the economic disparities in health care for different groups of women exposed the great challenges to successful cancer screening in a class-based society. Moreover, the whole nature of cancer surgery and the notion of radical operation seemed misogynistic. As Rose Kushner asked, why were women excluded from the decisions about treating their own bodies? It became clear that although women had defined the educational messages, they had been offered little input in determining treatment. After more than fifty years of volunteering time and energy to spread information about cancer throughout the United States, women were now demanding that they have a say in the diagnosis and treatment stage as well.

The groundswell of activism that emerged in this period recognized patient advocacy and legitimized experiential knowledge. To be sure, cancer activism had always privileged the patient's voice as an effective means to educating the public. Learning from this cue, female cancer survivors continued to employ the rhetoric of autobiography but used their personal experience as a way to challenge the medical system and inform public policy.

Conclusion

On December 22, 1973, one of the most popular shows on American television, *All in the Family*, aired "Edith's Christmas Story." This hour-long drama that centered on a family of four spelled out contemporary knowledge, treatment, and awareness of breast cancer. Edith, the mother of the family, sits alone in the kitchen with her daughter, Gloria. Edith suddenly blurts out, "I got a lump in my breast." "What?" Gloria asks, dumbfounded. "I got a lump in my breast," Edith repeats. As Gloria moves toward her mother and hugs her, Edith's voice cracks, and she whispers, "That's the first time I said it out loud."[102]

This 1973 episode reflected the expanding forum for public discussions of breast cancer and women's health concerns. The plot that evolved in this *All in the Family* episode captured several aspects of breast cancer in American culture in the 1970s. Significantly, it reflected the reticence many people felt about discussing certain aspects of the disease. Despite the publicity that surrounded the women's health movement, every woman faced individual concerns that defined a cancer experience. The peculiar situation and family dynamics in this show contextualized Edith's personal experience.

Edith explains to Gloria how she discovered the lump. After reading a magazine article about the breast self-examination, she performed one and recognized a lump in her breast. She consulted her doctor who urged her to see a surgeon. When Gloria asks Edith when she was planning to tell Archie (Edith's husband), Edith adamantly replies, "Never. And don't you tell him neither. No Gloria, your father has enough to think about. Don't say nothing to your father or Mike." Emphasizing her desire to keep her diagnosis private, she adds that she does not want Gloria to tell anyone.

Later, Edith confides in her best friend, Irene. She tells her about the lump and shares her concern that she might have to have "one of those operations." "I'm afraid if I have this operation Archie won't think of me in the same way," she worries. Irene tries to assure Edith that everything would be fine, but Edith insists, "You don't know

Irene." Irene answers, "That's just the point Edith, I do know. I know." Finally, Irene reveals why: "Six years ago." She continues, "And you see how Frank and I get along. It hasn't made one bit of difference in our marriage." Edith stares at Irene's chest. "Don't bother looking Edith," Irene says, "you can't tell."

By the time Edith is scheduled for surgery, her husband and son-in-law have learned about the lump. All four characters go to the hospital together. Archie turns to Edith before the surgery and says, "You're my wife no matter what happens." In the final moments of the show, the comedic tone of *All in the Family* is restored. Edith's lump is benign, but she remains immobile in a hospital bed, explaining to her family, "When they told me everything was all right I got so excited I jumped off the exam table and broke my ankle!" Edith's experience with breast cancer was short-lived. Yet, her fear of a cancer diagnosis, concern about mastectomy, and reluctance to tell others about her biopsy addressed many of the issues that women experienced when diagnosed with cancer.

Conclusion

Contemporary references to a history of silence that surrounded breast cancer are inaccurate. Since early in the twentieth century, women have taught each other about cancer symptoms, encouraged early detection, and contributed to the creation and distribution of cancer awareness pamphlets, films, billboards, and more. Throughout the twentieth century, public discussions of cancer have consistently included advice to women about detecting cancer warning signs, but as the years have passed, the dialogue has been expanded to include recommendations about treatment options, the recognition of cancer survivor networks, autobiographical narratives that reveal feelings of fear and anxiety, and powerful women's organizations that effectively influence public policy related to cancer. These efforts to promote cancer awareness suggest that the "history of silence" is a myth. For decades, women (and men) have talked and written publicly about cancer. In the process, they laid the groundwork for the contemporary women's health movement.

Why, then, is there a lapse in the collective memory about early cancer awareness programs? These programs convinced popular women's magazines to publish articles about cancer as early as 1913, collaborated with the General Federation of Women's Clubs in the 1930s in order to teach its millions of members about cancer awareness, and packed movie houses with viewings of *The Breast Self-Examination* in the 1950s. There has not been a void in the public discussion of female cancers. Rather, frequent descriptions of a history of silence reflect a metaphorical reference to the types of discussions that surrounded women and cancer throughout much of the twentieth century. Although cancer awareness activism has been a consistent part of twentieth-century American culture, until the 1970s and 1980s public dialogue about women and cancer did not utilize a vocabulary that challenged traditional medical practices. This project has demonstrated that women have historically been invested in cancer awareness, detection, and control, but the impact of their investment in terms of medical practice has changed over time.

During the feminist health movement and afterward, the burst of public conversations, autobiographies, and political commentaries about women and cancer offered alternative ways for women to discuss cancer. Female cancer survivors presented radical viewpoints and created new terms for cancer discussions that stemmed from a feminist dialogue created by and for women. Some of the most notable activists of this era, like Rose Kushner, Audre Lorde, and Barbara Ehrenreich, challenged audiences to reconsider popular perceptions of medical treatment and cancer. Moreover, effective lobbying groups, including the National Alliance of Breast Cancer Coalitions, Susan G. Komen Breast Cancer Foundation, and particularly the National Breast Cancer Coalition (NBCC), ensured that women would be represented in the political debates about cancer funding, research, and programming.[1]

Feminists challenged the medical profession in the 1970s more openly than ever before, critiquing its treatment of female patients and its insistence about the immediacy of cancer surgery and the type of treatment. Talking about cancer in ways that centered the experience on patients and survivors, Rose Kushner, for one, rejected the formal instructions of cancer advice literature that urged uncritical deference to physicians.[2] She openly expressed her outrage with the Halsted radical mastectomy and the one-step mastectomy. Kushner garnered attention for her critique in 1975 when she published her pathbreaking analysis of cancer treatment, *Breast Cancer: A Personal History and Investigative Report*. This book offered an intimate and personal account of her diagnosis and outlined her conflict with standard medical practices that ignored women's voices and defied logic.[3]

Five years later, Audre Lorde published her powerful *The Cancer Journals*, one of the most persuasive critiques of the medicalization of breast cancer. From the perspective of an African American lesbian, Lorde wrote eloquently about how her identity intersected with her diagnosis. She felt removed from much of the support afforded by cancer groups and medical staff, not least of all, the *Reach to Recovery* program, and she questioned the usefulness of breast prosthesis for recovery. She argued that this artificial part hid the effects of mastectomy from the public eye and obscured recognition of the startlingly high numbers of breast cancer survivors in America. She asked the reader to envision the image of all women who had ever had mastectomies joining together to form a "clan" of one-breasted women. She persuasively argued that this image could be the most effective tool for eliciting responses from politicians, physicians, and others.[4]

Most recently, feminist author and critic Barbara Ehrenreich published "Welcome to Cancerland: A Mammogram Leads to a Cult of Pink Kitsch,'" where she wrote, "To the extent that current methods of detection and treatment fail or fall short, America's breast-cancer cult can be judged as an outbreak of mass delusion, celebrating survivorhood by downplaying mortality and promoting obedience to medical protocols known to have limited efficacy." In this article, which engaged some readers and outraged others, Ehrenreich questioned the usefulness of contemporary breast cancer culture. Through the lens of her personal experience with the disease, she examined the familiarity of breast cancer in contemporary society, describing her frustration with the ubiquity of breast cancer paraphernalia. Pink ribbons, remembrance teddy bears, races and walks, she claimed, created a celebratory breast cancer culture. Within her critique of cancer culture, she exposed the fallacy of early detection rhetoric, a critique rarely articulated to such a large audience. As she wrote, "Even if foolproof methods for early detection existed, they would, at the present time, serve only as portals to treatments offering dubious protection and considerable collateral damage."[5]

Ehrenreich's conclusions speak to the legacy and longevity of breast cancer awareness in the twentieth-century United States and beyond. Since 1913, the dominant public discussion of cancer has been framed around rhetoric of early detection. Women's responsibility in detecting cancer has been particularly pronounced. Ehrenreich's frustration, like the criticism evident in many feminist health circles today, recognizes that early detection has a useful but limited impact. Ehrenreich urged the public to consider alternative frameworks for conceptualizing the risk that cancer poses and the treatment courses available.

While some praised the analysis in "Welcome to Cancerland," many readers were offended on a variety of levels. For some, Ehrenreich's article trivialized coping mechanisms—events, artifacts, routines—that have played meaningful roles in many survivors' lives and in their healing processes. For others, she seemed to lack an appreciation of the sentiments and goals that frame many survivors' rituals. As one reader wrote, "What she would not see––and what she did not see in the activities she scorns––is why we do this."[6] All that said, Ehrenreich exposed the myth of progress that has been perpetuated again and again in representations of cancer in modern American culture. For all the public discourse, the mortality rates from breast cancer have remained fairly consistent in recent decades. The American Cancer Society estimated that 215,990 new cases of breast cancer would be detected in women in 2004, and 40,110 women would die from the disease.[7]

The work by Kushner, Lorde, and Ehrenreich represents the significant shifts in the public discourse surrounding women and cancer since 1970. In the twenty-first century women have claimed control of that discourse and inserted stories of personal experiences that evoke political response.[8] Beyond individual activists, powerful breast cancer advocacy groups lobby for additional cancer research funding, outreach and awareness programs, and additional treatment centers for breast and cervical cancer. One of the most influential groups, the National Breast Cancer Coalition, effectively recruits conservative, moderate, and liberal politicians to its side, raises an enormous amount of money annually, and teaches its members about advocacy. Its goal is no less ambitious than "to eradicate breast cancer, the most common form of cancer among women in the United States."[9]

Today, female cancer awareness efforts are a visible part of popular American culture. On any given day, audiences might learn about new studies in breast and cervical cancer in a daily newspaper, on local television stations, in popular movies, on billboard signs, or in any of the various promotions for walks, runs, and rides that benefit cancer organizations. Additional information about female cancers is channeled to women through pamphlets on breast and cervical care, which are easily accessible in hospital lobbies, physicians' offices, and even in lingerie stores. Cards that describe a proper breast self-examination hang from showerheads in private homes, athletic clubs, and locker rooms in the Young Women's Christian Association. Political groups such as the NBCC urge women to write to Congress, sign petitions, and travel to Washington, D.C., for marches that advance women's health issues.

The history of women's participation in cancer awareness programs, evident since the early decades of the twentieth century, suggests its influence on the extraordinary changes of recent decades. Most notably, the emphasis on early detection, the primary message of cancer education as early as 1913, continues to serve as the dominant ideology in cancer activism today. Efforts to ensure that the message reaches all audiences of women, support for research that promises technological solutions for even earlier detection, and physician messages about compliance with suggested self-examinations show that the devotion to early detection resonates just as loudly today.

Early detection is a useful model and made an immeasurable positive impact on cancer survival rates throughout the twentieth century. The dramatic decline in uterine and cervical cancer rates since the introduction of the Pap smear offers a vivid example of its promise.[10] However, the continual rise in breast cancer incidence in the

United States, until very recently at least, should perhaps cause more people to wonder if this message is as useful as the propaganda implies. The urgency attached to the education message in the postwar years was ignited by a culture that was optimistic about the role of science and medicine in the future, certain that "experts" could eventually answer the riddle of cancer, and confident that all Americans, including women, would have access to health care. As we recognize the shortcomings of these expectations, it is important to reevaluate the message of early detection and recognize its position vis-à-vis cancer prevention, research, and treatment.

The message of blame in the postwar literature is also still evident in contemporary discussions of female cancers. Routinely, popular newspapers and magazines publish feature stories about a new study on female cancer. The results of the studies, while rarely conclusive, suggest that women adapt their lifestyle to decrease their risk of cancer by adjusting dietary regimens, alcohol consumption, exercise patterns, levels of stress, forms of birth control, sleeping patterns, vitamin supplements, and on and on. The popular press reports the finding that emphasizes how women should alter their behavior. Each reader processes the information differently, but clearly one way to make sense of the plethora of information is to assume that women's lifestyles in some way have played a role in their cancer diagnoses. In a recent "Dear Abby" column, for instance, a reader wrote, "I have a friend in her early 40s who is dying of cancer. 'Claire' had a Class II pap test years ago, but she never went back for a recheck." "Abby" offered her regret about the news and added, "the WORST is that because the patient procrastinated the condition has become so advanced that it's impossible to treat."[11] Although the emphasis on early detection is important, in columns such as these, the complications of cancer are glossed over and the impact of individual behavior may be overstated. Early detection does not guarantee survival, and late detection does not always lead to death. Abby's response also suggests that the woman bears the sole responsibility for her death and raises no concern for the variety of extenuating circumstances that may have framed her decision, including financial constraints, mistrust of the medical profession, and concerns about standard treatment.

Contemporary women's health activists who work to inform women about the importance of pelvic examinations and mammograms must remember that early detection is only one part of cancer diagnosis and treatment. More recent criticism by the renowned breast cancer surgeon Susan Love suggests that the emphasis on early detection may also be creating a false sense of security: "The harm is that they give us a false sense that we have a good way to find cancers and cure them and that very sense may keep us from redirecting resources to finding a better approach." In the mid-1990s Nancy Wartic and Julie Felner published similar sentiments in *Ms.*, suggesting that early detection fosters a psychological culture that teaches women to fear their bodies, particularly their breasts. As these scholars and activists suggest, emphasis on early detection has perhaps delayed political inquiry into other causal factors of cancer, such as the continual increase of toxins in the environment.[12]

Today, women's health activists have directed attention to other contributing factors to cancer incidence and mortality. Discussions about innovations in treatments specific to female cancers, the insistence that women be included in medical research trials, and advocacy for research that explores the causes of women's cancers embody this trend. Perhaps most significant, in the twenty-first century female volunteers and activists are working to increase funding for both detection and treatment centers at a steady rate, reflecting a new approach for cancer activism that is less dependent on the rhetoric of early detection. But as Ehrenreich's article reminds us, popular support programs do not have the same effect as political advocacy.

Throughout the twentieth century, formal networks of women have discussed women's susceptibility to cancer, informed women of early detection principles, and worked to decrease morbidity from this disease. As Barbara Clow has written, "Lay experience with conventional cancer therapies likewise shaped the health care choices of patients: information gleaned from family, friends, neighbors, and even the media could outweigh the advice offered by physicians and surgeons."[13] In addition to the formal networks fostered by the American Society for the Control of Cancer and the American Cancer Society, women have certainly learned about female cancers through informal networks of women, in private conversations with their mothers, sisters, and friends, in interactions with physicians, and in discussions about death and dying.

In the midst of recent and very successful efforts to redefine women's health and apply more resources and consideration to female cancers, this history has been overlooked. In the United States, grassroots efforts to educate women and promote cancer awareness have existed for nearly a century, and women have played central roles in these efforts. To be sure, cancer education has frequently targeted privileged audiences, yet these early efforts introduced popular discussions of cancer to diverse communities of women. In order to better understand the historical legacy of cancer activism, we must consider its implications.

Created by women, for women, and with women, early cancer education programs favored early detection. Cancer awareness, initially defined by medical professionals invested in promoting their profession, convinced audiences that early detection offered physicians the key to curing cancer. The faith we still place in early detection may be based as much on the nearly century-long crusade to reinforce this message to all Americans, as on its scientific merit. Without diminishing the usefulness of this message, as we enter the twenty-first century and consider the dramatic changes in cancer awareness, scientific knowledge, and treatment options, we may want to revisit alternative cancer concerns, including environmental factors that contribute to female cancers, the continued marginalization of some communities from standard health care, and the quality of life for cancer patients.

Notes

ABBREVIATIONS

AAUW Archives
American Association of University Women Archives, Washington, D.C.

ACS   American Cancer Society

ASCC   American Society for the Control of Cancer

BFP   Betty Ford Papers, President Gerald R. Ford Library, Ann Arbor, Mich.

BWHC   Boston Women's Health Collective

GFWC   General Federation of Women's Clubs

GFWC Archives
General Federation of Women's Clubs Archives, Washington, D.C.

LC   Manuscript Division, Library of Congress, Washington, D.C.

LCPP   Prints and Photographs Division, Library of Congress, Washington, D.C.

MLP   Mary Lasker Papers, Columbia University Rare Book and Manuscript Library, New York, N.Y.

NCNW Collection
National Council of Negro Women Collection, Mary McLeod Bethune House, Washington, D.C.

TBA   National Association for the Study and Prevention of Tuberculosis

WFA   Women's Field Army

YWCA   Young Women's Christian Association

1. As one example, Love and Lindsey, *Dr. Susan Love's Breast Book*, is currently in its fourth edition.
2. For the creation of the National Breast Cancer Coalition, see Stabiner, *To Dance with the Devil*. See also Grady, "In Breast Cancer Data, Hope, Fear, and Confusion."
3. Kolata, "Vying for the Breast Vote."
4. *National Breast Cancer Coalition*. See section entitled "Visions."
5. Batt, *Patient No More*, xiii.
6. Angier, "Confronting Cancer."
7. Clow, "Who's Afraid of Susan Sontag?" 297–98.
8. Adams, "What Can We Do about Cancer?"; "The Protection of Women from Cancer: An Educational Program by Women, for Women, with Women," January 12, 1931, 1, Box 4, Folder "Protection," Becker Papers, LC.
9. Reagan, "Engendering the Dread Disease."
10. Debates about the value of mammography began in the 1960s with its introduction. The debates became especially fierce in early 2000, as scientists reviewed and questioned the clinical trials that first legitimized mammography. See "What Is All the Fuss About?"
11. Previous studies on women's health activism show similar trends. Susan Smith's work on black women's health activism and Sandra Barney's work on Appalachian women's health offer two examples. Smith, *Sick and Tired of Being Sick and Tired*; Barney, *Authorized to Heal*.
12. The Harkin Amendment to the Fiscal Year 1993 Department of Defense Appropriation Act allocated $210 million to the U.S. Army to support breast cancer programs. This generated more support for breast cancer research than any other national agency, including the National Cancer Institute. See T. Harkin Department of Defense Appropriation Act; Kaiser, "Army Doles Out First $210 million"; and Schwartz, Slater, Heydrick, and Woollett, "AIBS News: A Report of the AIBS Peer-Review Process for the US Army's 1994 Breast Cancer Initiative."
13. Hoffman was a statistician and insurance agent who emphasized cancer's risk to "civilized" nations. While this effort was clearly motivated by certain financial benefits for insurance companies, Hoffman played a pivotal role in creating the first cancer society, directing attention to cancer early in the century, and defining cancer as the disease of the twentieth century. See "Dr. Hoffman Dies, Actuarial Expert." Francis J. Sypher is currently writing a biography of Hoffman and outlines many of Hoffman's achievements in a 2000 article for the Cosmos Club. See Sypher, "Rediscovered Prophet."
14. Medical specialists have also been instrumental in directing more attention, funding, and concern to cancer. Important to this story are practitioners who blurred the boundary between their professional role as doctors and their personal efforts to control this devastating disease. Several female physicians, including Drs. Catherine Macfarlane, Florence Rena Sabin, and Elise Strang L'Esperance, contributed to the ASCC/ACS early detection efforts.

15. Celebrities have often created the topics for news. As one commentator noted, "Television newswomen have been indispensable in transforming breast cancer from a source of private shame into a very public, very political crusade." See Orenstein, "Scheduling Breast Cancer in Prime Time." A celebrity's reaction to a cancer diagnosis often shaped popular images of cancer more powerfully than meticulously executed public education efforts. Betty Ford's reaction to her breast cancer diagnosis and mastectomy set this trend. Thousands of supportive letters poured into the White House revealing the intense sympathy of the American public for this diagnosis. Her willingness to discuss the disease directly inaugurated a new era for public discussion of female cancers that complemented the women's health movement. For more, see chapter 5.

16. As in Hoffman, *Some Essential Statistics of Cancer Mortality*, 8. Hoffman divided female cancers into two types—"female generative organs" or "female breast"—for his statistical charts for data from 1901 to 1913.

17. *Vital Statistics of the United States*, 24. In 1936–37 over 16,000 women died of uterine cancer, compared to the nearly 14,000 women who died of breast cancer. Ovarian cancer killed far fewer women, but it was the deadliest form of cancer, then and now.

18. I recognize that men compose 1 percent of breast cancer victims. This narrative focuses, however, on the 99 percent who are female victims of breast cancer. Also, beginning in 1913 the cancer education campaign frequently grouped a variety of female cancers under the title "reproductive cancers." Likewise, it often conflated uterine and cervical cancer. As one example, see ASCC, *Important Facts for Women about Tumors*, 9–12, where the description of uterine cancer includes within it a description of cervical cancer.

19. Reagan, "Engendering the Dread Disease." Reagan offers insight about how gender created distinct messages for men and women in cancer awareness campaigns.

20. Patterson, *Dread Disease*, 198–99. One example of postwar cancer research includes the ACS's funding of the Pap smear.

21. For a more extensive look at this issue, see Gardner, "Hiding the Scars"; and "From Cotton to Silicone."

22. Meyerowitz, *Not June Cleaver*.

23. Kentucky State File, *Records of the National Association of Colored Women's Clubs*, reel 21, frame 733. Thank you to Joan Johnson for locating this for me.

24. One manifestation of this concern was the production and distribution of Spanish-language films, posters, and pamphlets. For examples see ACS, *Atencion: Viva mas!*, and *Corra la voz acera de los Mamogramas*, LCPP; and *Luisa Tenia Razon*.

25. Ford with Chase, *Times of My Life*; and Ford with Chase, *Betty*.

26. A few examples of this work are Scott, *Natural Allies*; Higginbotham, *Righteous Discontent*; and Boylan, *Origins of Women's Activism*.

27. For example, see Clow, *Negotiating Disease*.

1. ASCC, *Facts about Cancer*.
2. Adams, "What Can We Do about Cancer?" Other than circulation records, it is hard to determine how many women read this article and how they responded to it. After writing to the magazine, I learned that *Ladies' Home Journal* does not have any archives open to the public. The magazine also admits that when it changed ownership in the mid-1960s, much of their archival material "disappeared because of the sale and moving around." Letter to the author, December 5, 1997.
3. Adams, "What Can We Do about Cancer?" 21. Samuel Hopkins Adams (1871–1958), a popular journalist and muckraker, wrote about the content of patent medications in 1905 and investigated conditions of public health throughout the early twentieth century. See Kennedy, *Samuel Hopkins Adams and the Business of Writing*.
4. Adams's reference to a "half-operation" warned readers against unorthodox cures and doctors who practiced outside of the American Medical Association. Often referred to as "quacks" in the early twentieth century, licensed M.D.s organized and delegitimized these practitioners. The ASCC joined these efforts.
5. Starr, *Social Transformation of American Medicine*; and Tomes, *Gospel of Germs*.
6. Tomes, *Gospel of Germs*; Apple, "Constructing Mothers."
7. Apple, "Constructing Mothers."
8. Tomes, *Gospel of Germs*, 113.
9. Ibid., 114–16.
10. ASCC, *Facts about Cancer*, 1.
11. Proctor, *Cancer Wars*, 16.
12. For additional examples, see Olson, *Bathsheba's Breast*.
13. Rather, "Johannes Müller," 1, 13, 27 (quotation). One of Müller's students, Rudolf Virchow, further explained cellular division and its role in tumor formation. As a pathologist, political activist, and physician, Virchow popularized contemporary theories in cellular pathology that recognized that abnormal cells derived from normal ones. His 1858 publication *Die Cellularpathologie in ihrer Begründung auf physiologische und pathologische Gewebenlehre* articulated the idea that over time, normal cells could transform into abnormal shapes and sizes, leading to tumor formation. He demonstrated that disease began in an individual cell that divided and spread over time. He inspired the field of histology, whereby scientists recorded patterns of tumor origins, growth, and behavior and recognized distinct cells that threatened the host. Histology allowed scientists to distinguish various tumors as "malignant" (life-threatening) or "benign" (less threatening). Finally, pathologists identified a pattern in malignant tumors whereby cancerous cells could spread and create secondary tumors, naming this process "metastases." See also "Johannes Müller," *Encyclopaedia Britannica Online*, <http://search.eb.com/eb/article-9054219> (January 14, 2004); and "Rudolf Virchow: Early Career" and "Rudolf Virchow: Medical

Investigations," *Encyclopaedia Britannica Online*, <http://search.eb.com/eb/article-9075460> (January 14, 2004).

14. Calatayud and González, "History of the Development and Evolution of Local Anesthesia," 1503. Dentists Horace Wells and William Thomas Green Morton gained notoriety for their use of ether as anesthesia in 1846. For a persuasive history of germ theory and its application to popular culture, see Tomes, *Gospel of Germs*.

15. Olson, *Bathsheba's Breast*, 45, 58–64; Lerner, *Breast Cancer Wars*, 17–28.

16. Halsted, "Results of Operations for the Cure of Cancer of the Breast," 297; Lerner, *Breast Cancer Wars*, 17–23.

17. Although Halsted traced historical cases, charting patients over multiple years, his statistics often obscured deaths after three years and from non-local recurrence. Contemporary evaluation of his statistics yields significantly different results than his summary findings.

18. Lerner, *Breast Cancer Wars*, 17–28; Olson, *Bathsheba's Breast*, 58–64. Halsted referred to his complete method as *en bloc* excision, which removed the breast, chest muscle, and/or axilla lymph nodes in one section.

19. Krementsov, *Cure*, 7.

20. Aronowitz, "Do Not Delay," offers details about physicians who supported the "do not delay" message and others who challenged this doctrine.

21. *American College of Surgeons Commission on Cancer*, 31.

22. Park, "Campaign against Cancer," 712.

23. Tomes, *Gospel of Germs*.

24. ASCC, "Facts about Cancer."

25. Several articles noted the similarity of the two organizations. As one example see "Surgeons Discuss Cancer Campaign," 509: "Within the limits of its special field and problems the work of the society will be somewhat analogous to that of the National Association for the Study and Prevention of Tuberculosis."

26. Cancer is a disease of longevity, and therefore its incidence increases as the average life span is extended. Throughout the early twentieth century, numerous popular articles suggested simple cause and effect scenarios to explain cancer. For example, "Relation of Beer to Cancer" or "Cancer and the Meat Eater" suggested that cancer could be controlled with minor lifestyle adjustments. Similarly, see "Lack of Light as a Prevalent Cause of Cancer." Likewise, strong opinions about cancer cures appeared with some frequency. "Experts" suggested everything from Finsen phototherapy to violet leaf treatment could cure cancer. "Curing Cancer by the Finsen Phototherapy System"; "Violet Leaf Treatment of Cancer."

27. Aronowitz, "Do Not Delay," 360–63. Aronowitz examines the medical opinions of Janet Lane-Claypon, James Ewing, and E. A. Daland, as well as the skepticism of surgeon Ian MacDonald.

28. Davis, *Fellowship of Surgeons*, 118; Coe, "Address of the President," 12–13.

29. Ross, *Crusade*, 20–21, 244.

30. Shaughnessy, "Story of the American Cancer Society," 22. The board of directors, however, remained 100 percent male until 1943, even though a 1936 "Report of the Managing Director to the Board of Directors" had suggested

that women be added to the board. For a sampling of Mead's participation in cancer control efforts through the years, see "Cancer Fund Is Drive Started in City"; "Celebrity Fete Tonight"; and "Charity Event Today at the Biltmore."

31. The charter members were Dr. James Ewing of the Association of Pathologists and Bacteriologists; Drs. Howard Taylor, Thomas Cullen, William E. Studdiford, and Frank F. Simpson of the American Gynecological Association; Drs. George Brewer, Joseph Bloodgood, C. L. Gibson, and Clement Cleveland of the American Surgical Association; Dr. S. Pollitzer of the American Dermatological Society; and John E. Parsons, George C. Clark, James Speyer, V. Everit Macy, and Thomas M. Debevoise. The physicians came from New York, Louisville, Baltimore, Boston, Philadelphia, Pittsburgh, New Orleans, and Denver. Ross, *Crusade*, 243–48; Shaughnessy, "Story of the American Cancer Society," 27.

32. "Control of Cancer," 840.

33. The American Medical Association House of Delegates endorsed the society in a spring 1913 vote. The Clinical Congress of Surgeons of North America pledged its support in a meeting on November 14, 1913. The Western Surgical Association and the Southern Surgical and Gynecological Association both endorsed the ASCC in 1913, at meetings in St. Louis and Atlanta, respectively. ASCC, *Facts about Cancer*, 2–3. The American Gynecological Society secured $5,000 for the first year of the ASCC. See "Report of the Committee on the Ways and Means in the Matter of Impressing Physicians and Educating the Public in the Necessity of Early Diagnosis and Operation in Cancer."

34. As historian Richard Shryock explained about early meetings of the TBA, "The need for emphasis on educational programs was apparent, and the members agreed that the public must be informed." Shryock, *National Tuberculosis Association*, 76.

35. See Tomes, *Gospel of Germs*; Shryock, *National Tuberculosis Association*; and Cameron, *Tuberculosis Medical Research*. Compared to other medical societies of the day, notably the TBA, the ASCC had a pitiful budget.

36. ASCC, *Certificate of Incorporation*, 1 (quotation); Patterson, *Dread Disease*, 71–78; Ross, *Crusade*, 15–22; ASCC, *American Society for the Control of Cancer: Its Objects*, 5–11. The central office was established in New York City, and the ASCC was officially incorporated in the state of New York on May 8, 1922. Ross, *Crusade*, 15–22.

37. Rigney, *History of the American Society for the Control of Cancer*, 12; "Rich Women Begin a War on Cancer."

38. Ross, *Crusade*, 20–21.

39. Throughout the 1920s–40s, prominent New York female philanthropists held card games, luncheons, theater shows, and more to raise funds for the ASCC. Most often, the hostesses' first names are absent, and instead the women are listed as Mrs. Francis J. Rigney, Mrs. Robert Mead, and Mrs. Samuel A. Clark. Gertrude Clark (Mrs. Samuel A. Clark) served for many years as the chair of social service at St. Luke's Hospital and routinely raised

money for cancer research. See "Mrs. S. A. Clark"; and "Street Fair in View for Needy Patients."

40. Hushberg, "How Cancer May Be Prevented," 11.

41. "Progress Hailed in Cancer Clubs."

42. ASCC, *Facts about Cancer*, 2. In addition to publicly identifying the elite and wealthy supporters of the organization, this circular recognized the volunteer labor that women donated to the society. These women had predecessors in Mrs. John Jacob Astor and Mrs. George W. Cullum, who founded Memorial Hospital for the treatment of cancer in 1884. Likewise, Mrs. Collis P. Huntington established the first cancer research fund in America. See ASCC, *There Shall Be Light!*

43. "Vanderbilts and the People of Hyde Park."

44. "Abby Aldrich Rockefeller, 1874–1948." In 1926 John D. Rockefeller Jr. made a donation of $100,000 to the ASCC for its Mohonk conference.

45. Mulhearn, "Women in Philanthropy."

46. Bloodgood, "Evidence of Value of Education in Cancer Control."

47. ASCC, *Cancer Control*, 163–64.

48. To be sure, some of the attention directed to cancer preceded the formation of the ASCC. Between 1900 and 1904 the *Readers' Guide* indexed thirteen articles about cancer; between 1905 and 1908 it indexed thirty-two articles under the subject "cancer"; and from 1909 to 1913 it listed seventy-three articles about cancer. Of the thirteen articles published between 1900 and 1904, four focused on cancer cures (phototherapy or radium), seven on the "cancer problem" (including statistics on the increasing incidence of cancer in America), and two on the causes of cancer. Later articles listed under the subject heading "cancer" also included explorations of potential cancer cures, theories about the cause of cancer, and statistical data on the disease. *Readers' Guide to Periodical Literature* (Vol. 1: 1900–1904), 219; (Vol. 2: 1905–1909), 340–41; (Vol. 3: 1910–1914), 401–2.

49. Bloodgood, "What Everyone Should Know about Cancer"; "Prevention and Cure of Cancer"; Hirshberg, "How Cancer May Be Prevented"; "Surgeons Discuss Cancer Campaign."

50. Curtiss Anderson, editor of *Ladies' Home Journal* in 1963, praised the magazine's publication record on the topic: "Fifty years ago, in May, 1913, the *Journal* published the first article on cancer ever to appear in a popular magazine, *What Can We Do about Cancer?* By Samuel Hopkins Adams." He described this editorial decision as "bold" and "life-saving." Lescher, "Painless New Way To Detect Breast Cancer," 13.

51. For a discussion of the significance of time in cancer awareness messages since 1900, see Aronowitz, "Do Not Delay."

52. Adams, "What Can We Do about Cancer?" 21. Although this article targeted women, public awareness efforts encouraged men to be mindful of early indications of cancer as well.

53. Ibid., 22.

54. Wiley, "*If* You *Think* You Have *a Cancer*." Wiley was also the person in charge of pure food and drug regulation.

55. Bloodgood, "Greatest Scourge in the World." See chapter 2 for more discussion of Bloodgood's role in cancer control. See also Patterson, *Dread Disease*, 91.

56. Wood, "Must Women Die of Cancer?" *Woman Citizen* was an organ of the League of Women Voters and targeted a different audience than popular women's magazines.

57. For a more detailed discussion of the expansion of the popular discussion of breast cancer since 1970, see chapter 5.

58. Hirshberg, "How Cancer May Be Prevented," 11.

59. "Facing Cancer with Courage," 421.

60. Aronowitz, "Do Not Delay."

61. Rima D. Apple makes a compelling argument about the rise of scientific motherhood in this period, which suggests similar trends in other movements for women's health in the early twentieth century. See Apple, "Constructing Mothers."

62. Wild, "Danger Signals of Cancer," 700.

63. Carnett, "Cancer of the Breast."

64. Aronowitz, "Do Not Delay."

65. "Easier Steps Are the Best First Steps," 899. By midcentury the "habit of periodically examining her own breast tissue" would be named the breast self-examination (BSE).

66. Adams, "What Can We Do about Cancer?" 22.

67. Carnett, "Cancer of the Breast," 262.

68. "I'm Not Afraid of Cancer," 140. Although a formal breast self-examination was not introduced into the cancer movement until the 1940s, frequent reference to women's ability to detect a lump implied some sort of visual or tactile examination.

69. Patterson, *Dread Disease*, 137–71.

70. Walker, *Women's Magazines*, 3–4.

71. ASCC, *American Society for the Control of Cancer: Its Objects*, 16.

72. "I'm Not Afraid of Cancer," 140.

73. "Cancer Campaign Planned."

74. *National Negro Health News* 1 (January/March 1933): 1. This first issue explained that this quarterly bulletin offered a place for announcements and data pertaining to National Negro Health Week.

75. "Negro Health Week to Begin April 5."

76. "Cancer Education Via Radio."

77. *Great Peril.* The film opens with a "List of Players": Alden Chase played Dr. Crane; Warren Cooke played Dr. Charles Crane (Gordon's father); Amy Dennis played Margaret Salter; Jane Jennings played Mrs. Salter; Harold Clarendon played Mr. Whythe; Joseph Bannon played his assistant, and Andrew Andruss played George Gwyn. I have been unable to locate production notes on this film sponsored by the ASCC. It is also unclear how many people viewed the film; nevertheless, the film does offer one reflection of how the ASCC dramatized the physician's role in cancer education, women's role in organizing lectures, and female cancer patients. Thanks to the ACS, which sent me a copy of this film.

78. ASCC, *American Society for the Control of Cancer: Its Objects*. See also "25,000 Hear Cancer Talk"; and "War against Cancer." These articles applaud clinics, lectures, radio programs, and more.

79. ASCC, *Important Facts for Women about Tumors*, 3.

80. For example, in 1929 "What Every Woman Should Do about Cancer" was translated into "Jewish, French, Italian, Russian, Slovak, and Polish," according to Rigney, *History of the American Society for the Control of Cancer*, 44.

81. ASCC, *Important Facts for Women about Tumors*, 5.

82. Ibid., 5.

83. Ibid., 11.

84. Ibid., 12.

85. Ibid., 15. As explained in this booklet, "Lack of funds need not discourage a patient from seeking competent medical service. All physicians of recognized ability give due consideration to the financial situation of the patient; and all reputable medical hospitals regulate their charges accordingly."

86. ASCC, *Cancer Control*, 1.

87. Barney, *Authorized to Heal*; Smith, *Sick and Tired of Being Sick and Tired*.

88. ASCC press release, March 10, 1931, AAUW Archives; "Cheatle Endorses Three Cancer Aids"; "Spread of Cancer Greatest in Men."

89. The American Medical Association issued a series of pamphlets that warned the public about "quacks" in the 1920s. See the Historic Health Fraud Collection, American Medical Association Archives, Chicago, for numerous examples, including "Cancer Cures and Treatments," Box 467, Folder 0467-10.

90. Between 1920 and 1930, cancer moved from the third- to second-leading cause of death. Patterson, *Dread Disease*, 95.

91. "11,600 Cancer Cases Aided by Group Here"; "Charity Event Today at the Biltmore"; "Dinner to Aid Education."

92. Congress expanded the Marine Hospital Service into the U.S. Public Health Service in 1912. The department had limited power, and its budget did not include any specific funds for cancer research. Legislation by Congress in 1922 broadened the work of the U.S. Public Health Service and specifically included the control of cancer as a public health program. Williams, *United States Public Health Service*; Rettig, *Cancer Crusade*; Starr, *Social Transformation of American Medicine*.

93. 70th Cong., 1st sess., *Congressional Record* 69 (May 18, 1928): 9049–50.

94. Ibid., 9050. On Neely see *Who's Who in America: 1938–1939*, 1845. After Neely introduced the bill, the press gave it enough attention to generate the thousands of letters he received. The bill was not passed.

95. 70th Cong., 1st sess., *Congressional Record* 69 (May 18, 1928): 9049–50.

96. Ibid., 9050.

97. Patterson, *Dread Disease*, 88–92.

98. Ibid., 90.

99. This conclusion is based on a review of the *Congressional Record* and all discussions indexed under "cancer" in this era.

100. "Report of the Surgeon General," 272–74.
101. Ibid., 272 (emphasis in original).
102. Ibid., 273.
103. Ibid., 273.
104. Ibid., 274.
105. Bland, "Cancer in Women," 460.
106. Hoffman, *Some Cancer Facts and Fallacies*, 9.

CHAPTER TWO

1. Wheeling, West Virginia, Department of Vital Statistics has no death records for Amanda Sims. Response from June 2002 inquiry.
2. Lerner, "Fighting the War on Breast Cancer." Lerner traces the history of military rhetoric in cancer control campaigns, especially those campaigns that targeted breast cancer. For a sample of war rhetoric see "New Basis Urged for War on Cancer"; "War on Cancer Pressed: Women Are Urged to Enlist in Field Army This Week"; "Widen War on Cancer"; and "Attack on Cancer Likened to War."
3. This idea of "middling figure" is inspired by Nancy Hunt's work on colonial medicine in the Congo. See Hunt, *Colonial Lexicon of Birth Ritual, Medicalization, and Mobility*.
4. Women had a history of supporting various health crusades and education campaigns, including work for tuberculosis and other diseases. As one example, see Ott, *Fevered Lives*.
5. Becker to Loder, April 9, 1932, Florence Deakins Becker Papers, LC. Although I have searched numerous archives and newspapers for additional information on Amanda Sims, I have been unable to determine what type of cancer caused her death.
6. Joseph Colt Bloodgood (1867–1935) received his M.D. from the University of Pennsylvania in 1891. He served as resident physician at Philadelphia's Children's Hospital in 1891–92 and then moved to Johns Hopkins University for the remainder of his career. See *Who Was Who in America*, 1:76, 109. He published hundreds of articles, many dealing with cancer. See Bloodgood and Long, *Index to the Writings of Joseph Colt Bloodgood*.
7. 70th Cong., 1st sess., *Congressional Record* 69 (May 18, 1928): 9050; Patterson, *Dread Disease*, 88–90.
8. Perhaps due to the limited funds, Bloodgood chose this small, at-risk population as his primary beneficiary. Bloodgood's gynecology experience convinced him that significant progress in curing cervical cancer could be made if physicians treated the vaginal tears that resulted from childbirth and monitored their healing. He stressed that many cases of cervical cancer developed from these minor injuries and urged their immediate repair to prevent the onset of cancer. Like most cancer experts of this era, Bloodgood believed that cancer in its earliest stage was small, localized, and effectively treated with surgery. He endorsed postnatal medical care, including routine,

semiannual pelvic examinations, as an effective and practical way to begin prevention screening for cervical cancer.

9. "Biographical Information," Becker Finding Aid, Becker Papers, LC. After her divorce from Forrester, Becker used the name Mrs. George F. Becker or Florence Deakins Becker.

10. Becker to Matheson, February 24, 1931, Box 4, Folder "G–M," Becker Papers, LC.

11. See Joseph Bloodgood to Frank Pinneo, November 24, 1933, Folder "C–E," Becker Papers. Bloodgood wrote, "Mrs. Becker is rewriting my statements for women and has improved them greatly."

12. Bloodgood decided to direct this money and the educational effort to cervical cancer because he perceived this disease to be one of the most neglected female cancers. Although his educational efforts often included information about breast cancer and he continually advocated early detection of it, he believed breast cancer was already given much attention by the medical profession and the ASCC. The 1933 ASMF annual report defined Florence Becker's job as "Directress and Librarian." Bloodgood to Norbeck, n.d., Folder "Bloodgood," Becker Papers, LC (announcing Becker will temporarily take charge of the fund); "Report to Mr. Bloodgood," 1, Box 4, Folder "Cancer," Becker Papers, LC. On the medicalization of childbirth, see Martin, *Woman in the Body*.

13. Becker to Winifred, February 24, 1931, Box 4, Folder "G–M," Becker Papers, LC.

14. Bloodgood, "Cancer of the Cervix,"1241.

15. Bloodgood was a leading advocate of this idea. To be sure, female physicians also insisted that this message be spread. For example, Drs. Elise L'Esperance and Catherine Macfarlane supported efforts to teach more women about cancer.

16. Bloodgood recommended a semiannual exam for women over forty years of age and an annual exam for women under forty. See Bloodgood, "Cancer Prevention," 221. Bloodgood (through Becker's education program) was not advocating regular vaginal smears for indication of precancerous cells. This test, commonly referred to as the "Pap" smear, was not popularized until the 1950s.

17. Obstetricians and gynecologists created an exclusive specialization in 1930. At this time, many cancer advocates, most notably Bloodgood, urged regular annual exams. In the 1930s the military standard for female patients began to include routine gynecological exams. It is difficult to determine the percentage of women who complied with such guidelines, however. Bloodgood explained, "there is no question that in spite of fifteen years of educational efforts, less than ten percent are having their periodic pelvic examinations." The percentage of the entire female population who underwent exams was certainly even smaller. Bloodgood, "Purpose of Preventative Medicine," 2, Becker Papers, LC. See also Starr, *Social Transformation of American Medicine*, 356–57.

18. Bloodgood to McHale, October 14, 1931, AAUW Archives. Bloodgood frequently made assumptions based on gender. In this example, he assumed

a "young mother" would be uncomfortable and not open to a presumably male doctor. A more obvious example was his belief that "no beautiful woman suffers from cancer of the skin because she pays immediate attention to any skin blemish." Bloodgood, "Cancer Prevention," 220.

19. Letter dated March 23, 1931, Box 3, Folder "Bloodgood," Becker Papers, LC.

20. It is unclear why Becker and Bloodgood started their own educational effort instead of collaborating with the ASCC. Perhaps they were frustrated by the society and eager to begin an independent effort that was not shaped by the emerging bureaucracy of the ASCC. Bloodgood was likely critiquing the ASCC when he claimed that, despite the medical societies' efforts, "at the present moment the results of the education effort upon both the public and the profession of medicine lag behind chiefly in cancer of the cervix." See Bloodgood, "What Every Doctor, Dentist or Physician Should Know about Cancer," 9, Bloodgood Papers, Alan Mason Chesney Medical Archives, Johns Hopkins University, Baltimore, Md. Perhaps, too, Becker and Bloodgood wanted to begin a separate movement to recognize John Sims's donation for research on female cancers. Most likely, however, an independent movement allowed Becker and Bloodgood the freedom to focus on cervical cancer, a topic of special interest to Bloodgood. Bloodgood was clearly aware of the ASCC's efforts to educate the public about cancer in general. He was one of the society's fifteen founding members, supported its work, and served as a medical advisor and spokesperson for many of its publications. James Patterson's observation that the ASCC was limited to medical circles in these years might also explain this decision. Patterson, *Dread Disease*, 72. Perhaps Bloodgood and Becker's focus on laypersons could not be accommodated by the ASCC.

21. Bloodgood to McHale, February 21, 1931, AAUW Archives.

22. The meeting took place at the home of Mrs. Delos A. Blodgett. I spoke with Blodgett's daughter-in-law, who confirmed Blodgett's participation in philanthropic organizations, but she could not offer any particulars on Blodgett's cancer philanthropy. Telephone interview with the author, April 1998.

23. I first found this document in the Becker Papers, LC. Later searches for information on the document and its contents unearthed copies in the Bloodgood Papers, Alan Mason Chesney Medical Archives, Johns Hopkins University, Baltimore, Md.; the AAUW Archives; and in bound volumes of Bloodgood's reprinted papers at Johns Hopkins University. There are several reprints and editions of the letter, and the number of pages it included varies according to edition. The primary author was probably Joseph Bloodgood. Several references to "I" in the document referred to other publications that he authored and ideas he championed. I believe that Florence Becker surely had an enormous influence on this document also.

24. Aronowitz, "Do Not Delay."

25. "Reprint No. 335," *Protection of Women from Cancer*, 11, dated January 12, 1931, Box 4, Folder "G–M," Becker Papers, LC.

26. "Report to Dr. Bloodgood, 1933," Folder "Cancer," Becker Papers, LC. The report traces the educational programs, noting the 860 reprints sent to la-

ity. This movement, and most women's clubs of the era, included mainly white, middle- and upper-class women, although some of the clubs that participated in the movement, such as the YWCA, included a broader social spectrum. Although the Kentucky Division of the WFA started a "Colored Division" in 1939, I have no indication that this 1930s cervical cancer education movement included African Americans or other racial minority groups. "Mrs. Alice B. Crutcher," Kentucky State File, *Records of the National Association of Colored Women's Clubs*, reel 21, frame 733. See Smith, *Sick and Tired of Being Sick and Tired* for an insightful examination of African American women's health in the twentieth century. Smith's study notes very little on cancer activism. See chapter 4 for a discussion of the alliance that formed between the National Council of Negro Women and the ACS in 1960.

27. Becker to McHale, February 5, 1931, Box 101, Folder 14, AAUW Archives.

28. McHale to Bloodgood, February 11, 1931, Box 101, Folder 14, AAUW Archives. Bloodgood's article, "Cancer Prevention," appeared in the June 1932 issue of the *Journal of the American Association of University Women*. McHale was prepared to publish the article earlier, but Bloodgood did not write it until later.

29. For a thorough history of the American Association of University Women in the twentieth century, see Levine, *Degrees of Equality*, esp. 23–53. Levine's work also includes limited biographical information on McHale.

30. McHale to Bloodgood, February 11, 1931, Box 101, Folder 14, AAUW Archives.

31. Ibid.

32. Ibid. Information was the key ingredient to a successful public health campaign. As Nancy Tomes has argued, public health campaigns proved effective when they taught the public about germs and the scientific premise of bacteriology. Tomes, *Gospel of Germs*. In a different example, other early twentieth-century health campaigns, largely influenced by notions of race and ethnicity, failed to consider the value of patient education. See, for example, Leavitt, *Typhoid Mary*, and the confusion that Mary Mallon experienced as one of the first carriers of typhoid.

33. McHale to Bloodgood, February 11, 1931, Box 101, Folder 14, AAUW Archives. McHale's initial enthusiasm is evident in the numerous letters exchanged in February 1931. As she wrote about Bloodgood's article and his promise to help create a health education syllabus, "The more I think about the two possibilities, the more enthusiastic I become. The latter suggests unlimited educational opportunity in that we have a wide sale and distribution of our materials in adult education and that offers a new departure of need and value." McHale to Bloodgood, February 21, 1931, AAUW Archives.

34. *Journal of the American Association of University Women* 25, no. 1 (October 31, 1932): 48.

35. Becker to McHale, September 4, 1931, Folder "ASCC," AAUW Archives.

36. Bloodgood, "Cancer Prevention," 219, 220. See also *Journal of the American Association of University Women* 26, no. 2 (January 1933): 105.

37. American Association of University Women, *The Health of Women from Adolescence through Adulthood*, AAUW Archives.

38. As one example, Bloodgood funded McHale's visit to the Canadian Medical Society in the summer of 1931 so that she could share with audiences in the work of the American Association of University Women on cancer education. Becker to McHale, September 8, 1931, and McHale to Becker, September 9, 1931, Folder "ASCC," AAUW Archives.

39. Becker to Mrs. Smith, May 5, 1931, AAUW Archives. Within the next few years, the General Federation of Women's Clubs prioritized cancer education as a primary goal. It is unclear if the ASMF influenced this decision or not. Likewise, aside from the American Association of University Women, it is unclear how many women's groups responded to this cervical cancer awareness program for mothers.

40. The term "women's health" was not used in the 1930s; however, the ASMF movement reflected its principal components, including a woman-centered dialogue, recognition of patient experience, and an emphasis on education.

41. Bloodgood, "Cancer Prevention," 219. Bloodgood often cited the American Association of University Women in his published articles. For example, "Among all the national organizations of women in this country the American Association of University Women has done more to help disseminate correct information to mothers than any other." Bloodgood, "Cancer of the Cervix," 1245.

42. Becker to McHale, October 14, 1931, AAUW Archives.

43. Bloodgood and Becker eagerly embraced the notion of extending this movement beyond the borders of the United States. For example, after McHale received an invitation to address the Canadian Medical Society, Becker forwarded a personal check from Bloodgood for $75 to cover McHale's travel expenses. Becker admired Bloodgood's personal dedication to the cause, stating that "this is only an example of Dr. Bloodgood's unselfish and magnificent generosity towards assisting to protect the lives of women from developing cancer by correct information." Becker to McHale, September 8, 1931, AAUW Archives. After the initial embarrassment of accepting Dr. Bloodgood's personal check and several exchanges of correspondence, McHale learned that Bloodgood's personal funds kept the educational campaign and the ASMF financially solvent. McHale responded on September 9, 1931, explaining, "I infer from your letter that this is his personal check. I am a little embarrassed over this for the reason that his original suggestion to me was that . . . the money would come from that fund [the Amanda Sims Memorial Fund]." Becker then sent McHale a copy of the financial support for the ASMF, which indicated Bloodgood's contributions in excess of $1,000. Becker explained, "You will see that the funds have long since been exhausted, and that they have been carried on largely by Dr. Joseph Colt Bloodgood." McHale to Becker, September 9, 1931, and Becker to McHale, September 10, 1931, AAUW Archives. After meeting with the officers of Canadian Federation of University Women and the president of the National Council of Women of Canada, McHale reported that all

participants expressed excitement about the educational effort but wanted to gain support from the Canadian minister of health before launching any activities. McHale to Bloodgood, August 29, 1931, AAUW Archives.

44. Becker to Matheson, January 24, 1931, Box 4, Folder "G–M," Becker Papers, LC.

45. Becker to Acton, January 24, 1931, Box 2, Folder "A–B," Becker Papers, LC. On Acton, see *India Office List for 1932*, 493. Very few Indian women ever went to a physician. Only sophisticated, elite women with reform-minded families would go to a physician.

46. Bilhuber to Ahlers, July 22, 1932, AAUW Archives.

47. Marjorie Illig to "Health Chairmen," October 16, 1934, Box 4, Folder 0712088-5-4, GFWC Archives.

48. "THE NATION'S WOMANHOOD MUST DEFEND THE NATION'S HEALTH," Program Records, 1932–35, Box 4, Folder 712088-5-3, GFWC Archives. In this memo Illig also reminded members, "IT IS YOUR RESPONSIBILITY."

49. Clarence Cook "Pete" Little became director of the ASCC in 1929. An expert in genetics, a graduate of Harvard University, the former president of both University of Michigan and University of Maine, he also ran the Roscoe B. Jackson Memorial Laboratory in Bar Harbor. See Patterson, *Dread Disease*, 121; Ross, *Crusade*, 29.

50. "GFWC Annual Report, 1932–1933," 6, Box 4, Folder 0712088-5-5, GFWC Archives.

51. "Annual Report of the Division of Public Health, General Federation of Women's Clubs, 1933–1934," Box 4, Folder 0712088-5-5, GFWC Archives.

52. "Cancer Education Program," 1, Box 4, Folder 0712088-3-2, D-1a, GFWC Archives.

53. "Annual Report of the Division of Public Health, General Federation of Women's Clubs, 1933–1934," 5.

54. "Report of the Director of Public Health, 1932–1935," 3 (see subheading "Cancer Education Program"), Box 4, Folder 0712088-5-5, GFWC Archives.

55. *Health Programs of the National Women's Organizations* (New York: American Social Hygiene Association, publication no. A-7, n.d. [ca. 1936?]), 2, Box 4, Folder 0712088-5-2, GFWC Archives. See subheading "The General Federation of Women's Clubs."

56. "Annual Report, 1932–1933," 6, Box 4, Folder 0712088-5-5, GFWC Archives; Wells, *Unity in Diversity*, 226.

57. "Volunteer Group Drives on Cancer."

58. Patterson, *Dread Disease*, 122–23. Marjorie Illig served as the public health chair for the GFWC from 1932 to 1938. See Wells, *Unity in Diversity*, 226; and Patterson, *Dread Disease*, 122–24.

59. Poole was named the honorary national commander of the WFA after she retired from the GFWC presidency. For additional information on Grace Morrison Poole, see Wells, *Unity in Diversity*, 98–104.

60. Ibid., 226–27.

61. "Volunteer Group Drives on Cancer."

62. ASCC, *There Shall Be Light!* back cover.

63. Lerner, *Breast Cancer Wars*.

64. "Women's Field Army," 51–52; *Health Programs of the National Women's Organizations*, 3. According to "Campaign against Cancer," 117, "Every woman is eligible to membership and men may join as contributing members." Although WFA membership was limited to women, men assumed positions on the advisory boards for the organization.

65. For a discussion of military rhetoric and cancer, see Lerner, "Fighting the War on Breast Cancer."

66. ASCC, *Women's Field Army*; copy in Erskine Papers, E W842a, Masonic Grand Lodge Library, Cedar Rapids, Iowa.

67. Patterson, *Dread Disease*, 122–23; Ross, *Crusade*, 30–34. In 1945 the ASCC was renamed the American Cancer Society. One of the changes this introduced was the gradual absorption of the auxiliary WFA into the ACS. This started gradually, and by 1951 the office of the national commander had been discontinued.

68. The GFWC Division of Public Health was designed to promote health education among its members. "It has consistently been the policy to construct the program so that it will tie in with existing program activities of national, state, and municipal medical and health agencies." The GFWC sponsored programs as diverse as social hygiene, cancer education, public health nursing, tuberculosis control, mental hygiene, and recreation. See "The General Federation of Women's Clubs," in *Health Programs of the National Women's Organizations*, 1–2.

69. Ibid., 3; Marjorie Illig to Health Chairmen, October 16, 1934, Box 4, Folder 0712088-5-4, GFWC Archives. Illig referred to the "Healthward-Ho" program, an effort by the GFWC between 1932 and 1935 for the "protection and promotion of the health standards of our nation, states, and communities." This program encouraged collaboration between the GFWC and local and national health agencies. See also "Annual Report of the Division of Public Health, General Federation of Women's Clubs, 1933–1934," 1, Box 4, Folder 0712088-5-5, GFWC Archives.

70. "Cancer Education Program," 1–2, Box 4, Folder 0712088-5-2, GFWC Archives.

71. "Cancer Group Opens Booths for Recruits." The NYCCC hosted fourteen recruitment booths under the direction of Ella Rigney.

72. *There Shall Be Light!* 1.

73. Ibid.

74. Ibid. See also "Mrs. C. P. Huntington's Gift."

75. *There Shall Be Light!*

76. Similarly, the ASCC and NYCCC honored female M.D.s for their contributions to cancer control. Dr. Catherine Macfarlane won the Lasker Award in 1951; Dr. Elise L'Esperance won the Clement Cleveland Medal for cancer control work in 1942 and also won the Lasker Award in 1951; and Dr. Florence Rena Sabin was elected to the ASCC board of directors in 1943. See "Bi-Yearly Cancer Examinations"; "Cleveland Cancer Medal Awarded"; and "New Director Elected."

77. "There Shall Be Light!," 15.

78. ASCC, *There Shall Be Light*, 19.

79. Ibid., 5. The ASCC had established five offices near New York City by 1936, in Manhattan, Brooklyn, Forest Hills, Mineola, and Amityville.
80. 75th Cong., 1st sess., *Congressional Record* 81 (June 11, 1937): 5629.
81. 75th Cong., 1st sess., *Congressional Record* 81 (June 8, 1937): 5412. Bone, an attorney, was elected as a Democrat to the Senate in 1932 and reelected in 1938. "Homer Truett Bone."
82. 75th Cong., 1st sess., *Congressional Record* 81 (June 11, 1937): 5629. Rogers was elected to the Sixty-ninth Congress to replace her husband, John Jacob Rogers, after his death. She was reelected and to seventeen more Congresses, serving between 1925 and 1960. "Edith Nourse Rogers."
83. 75th Cong., 1st sess., *Congressional Record* (June 11, 1937): 5629. Although Nourse Rogers had supported cancer control efforts for much of her career, her obituary failed to note this work. A few days after the obituary appeared, one reader wrote, "However, one facet of her many humanitarian efforts was not touched upon. It was her tireless efforts on behalf of the nation's health, particularly cancer control. Mrs. Rogers was a pioneer in the American Cancer Society Women's Field Army. She served on its National Executive Council and was named Honorary National Commander in 1943." See "Tribute to Mrs. Rogers."
84. 75th Cong., 1st sess., *Congressional Record* 81 (July 30, 1937): 7915.
85. Aronowitz has written about several cancer critics of the era, including surgeon Ian MacDonald. See Aronowitz, "Do Not Delay."
86. Mary Hastings Bradley was a popular writer and journalist. She published over thirty books, and throughout the 1930s and 1940s she wrote articles for *McCall's*, *Cosmopolitan*, *Saturday Evening Post*, *Redbook*, *Ladies' Home Journal*, *Collier's*, and more. She also wrote popular children's books. Incidentally, her daughter Alice Bradley Sheldon also became a prolific writer, publishing under the pseudonym James Tiptree Jr. See <http://www.qinformation.com/Academic/Book/BookDisplay.asp?BookKey=408436> (October 25, 2005).
87. Bradley, *Pattern of Three*, 258.
88. Ibid., 259.
89. The publisher ran several advertisements in 1937 to publicize this new book. The advertisements focused on the dramatic narrative and offered no clues about how cancer propelled the plot. For example, see Display Ad 196 "Weekly News of Books," *New York Times*, January 9, 1938.
90. Bradley, *Pattern of Three*, 272. Eve's reference to Aunt Margaret, who presumably died of breast cancer, indicates that women might also have learned about the disease through family members.
91. *Choose to Live*.
92. Until the 1970s, if a woman had a breast biopsy that proved malignant, her breast would be amputated before she awoke from the surgery. This was referred to as a one-step mastectomy versus the more common procedure today, which is a two-step mastectomy that allows women to learn of the diagnosis before surgery.
93. Bix, "Disease Chasing Money and Power."
94. 75th Cong., 3d sess., *Congressional Record* 83 (February 9, 1938): 1739.

CHAPTER THREE

1. Patterson, *Dread Disease*, 171.
2. Evans, *Born for Liberty*, 219–41.
3. "War on Cancer Pressed: Women Urged to Continue Efforts Despite World Conflict."
4. "Post-War Control of Cancer Is Urged."
5. See Whitfield, *Culture of the Cold War*.
6. Cowan, *Social History of American Technology*, 310–18.
7. Mary Lasker was married to public relations expert Albert Lasker. She therefore had access to other public relations experts, most notably those who worked for the advertising agency Foote, Cone & Belding.
8. Mary Lasker interview transcript, Mary Lasker Oral History Project, Oral History Research Collection, Columbia University, New York, N.Y. See also Ross, *Crusade*.
9. Edwin MacEwan to Mary Lasker, February 18, 1946, Folder "ACS 1946," MLP.
10. To be sure, women doctors, such as Elise L'Esperance of New York City, Catherine Macfarlane of Philadelphia, and Augusta Webster of Chicago, also urged periodic cancer exams. See "Women Specialists on Cancer Confer."
11. Information on Mary Lasker can be found in MLP. The collection is large, containing 797 boxes. The ninety-two-page finding aid includes a personal narrative that Lasker wrote about major events in her life. This narrative explains that she had personal reactions to the devastating consequences of cancer and also observed how the disease affected others' lives. She became committed to the idea of controlling/curing cancer by midcentury.
12. Rettig, *Cancer Crusade*; Patterson, *Dread Disease*, 172–74.
13. Mary Lasker interview transcript, 151. Lasker recalled this memory nearly half a century later, and the dialogue is likely informed by her contemporary concern for cancer.
14. Ibid., section D. In addition, she lost a friend to cancer in 1928, and her husband, Albert Lasker, died from the disease in 1952. All of these events contributed to her dedication to cancer research and control.
15. Ibid., 106.
16. Ibid., 109.
17. Reinhardt had trouble with alcoholism throughout his adult life. This would eventually contribute to Mary's decision to divorce him.
18. Lasker's involvement in cancer activism would ultimately continue until her death and include restructuring the ASCC, coordinating aggressive political lobbying for increased research support, and personal significant financial contributions to cancer research.
19. Keenan, "Albert Davis Lasker."
20. Mary Lasker interview transcript, section titled "Our Role in the Development of the ACS and Its Support."
21. "Notes on the Development of the American Cancer Society's Campaigns for 1945 and 1956," Folder "Cancer—American Cancer Society 1946 Campaign," MLP.

22. Mary Lasker Interview Transcript, 477, MLP.
23. 1962 dinner notes, Box 78, MLP.
24. "Cancer, General, 1945," Box 75, MLP.
25. "1947," Boxes 75 and 76, MLP.
26. "ACS Reorganization Dated 5-2-45," Box 93, MLP. See also "ACS Details," Box 93, MLP, for a diagram of the reorganization and tiers of membership.
27. Mary Lasker interview transcript.
28. Patterson, *Dread Disease*, 173.
29. "Cancer—ACS 1946 Campaign," MLP.
30. "Cancer—General, 1944," Box 75, MLP. On November 9, 1946, Lois Mattox Miller was nominated to join the board of the New York City Cancer Committee.
31. Lois Mattox Miller to Emerson Foote, July 25, 1944, Box 75, Folder "Cancer, General, 1944," MLP.
32. "Notes on Development," 3, Box 75, Folder "Cancer—General 1946," MLP.
33. Mary Lasker interview transcript.
34. "Notes on Development," 3–5, Box 75, Folder "Cancer—General 1946," MLP.
35. Ibid. Albert Lasker and his sisters had donated $50,000 to the ASCC when their brother died from cancer. They stipulated that this money be used for cancer education publications.
36. Mary Lasker interview transcript, 488.
37. "We Could Cure Cancer Now!" 35. See also Patterson, *Dread Disease*, esp. chap. 6, "Hymns to Science and Prayers to Gods."
38. Patterson, *Dread Disease*, 140.
39. *Hygeia*, June 1945, 89.
40. Chemotherapy started after World War II with an accidental discovery that mustard gas also destroyed cancer cells.
41. Marshino, "Breast Cancer," 177.
42. See Reagan, "Engendering the Dread Disease," for a comparative analysis of cancer awareness programs for men and for women.
43. Starr, *Social Transformation of American Medicine*.
44. Holmes, "I Didn't Have Cancer"; Flexner, "Cancer—I've Had It," 57; Palmer, "I Had Cancer"; Lerner, *Breast Cancer Wars*, 87.
45. Flexner, "Cancer—I've Had It." Although they share a last name, Marion Flexner bore no relation to the renowned Abraham Flexner.
46. Ibid.
47. Ibid., 150.
48. Hellman, "Mary Roberts Rinehart." Rinehart began writing in the 1900s after her physician-husband lost money in the stock market. She continued writing after erasing the debt and after his death in 1931. By 1946 she was author of over fifty-seven books; Rinehart earned millions of dollars and ranked as one of the best-selling authors throughout her career.
49. Palmer, "I Had Cancer."
50. Ibid., 153.
51. Ibid., 152.
52. Ibid., 153; "Breast Self-Examination," 3.

53. "Alfred Marion Popma."

54. Ross, *Crusade*, 96–97. Leslie Reagan provided a thoughtful analysis of breast self-examination films at the 1998 conference "Women, Science, and Medicine in Postwar North America." "Projecting Breast Cancer" noted the different messages presented to physicians and to lay female audiences.

55. *Life Saving Fingers*. The film was produced in 1947 and gained copyright the next year. The Library of Congress has very limited reference information on this film. I interviewed Dr. Popma's daughter, Anne Frances Parsell, on June 28, 2000, about her memories of the film production. Although she was only in fourth grade at the time, she recalled that her father had people over for business, and they would use the bedroom. She peeked in the keyhole to see a woman with a bare chest. Apparently, when Mrs. Popma first saw the film, she recognized her own photograph on the bureau. Parsell also related that the woman who volunteered to conduct the breast self-examination was a professional model and the daughter of a cancer victim. Finally, she recalled one evening when her father showed the film to a group of Flying Fisherman in Idaho, who insisted that their wives view the film.

56. Interview with Anne Frances Parsell, June 28, 2000; Ross, *Crusade*, 96–97. The ACS recognized the significance of this film in 1989 when it embedded a copy of the film within the cornerstone of its newly constructed headquarters. See "Alfred Marion Popma."

57. The Film Division of the Library of Congress has an original reel of *Life Saving Fingers* that contains the label and an instruction sheet for viewing.

58. *Cancer: The Problem of Early Diagnosis*. This thirty-two-minute film stresses the value of early detection and outlines common symptoms, examination procedures, and treatment options for each of the cancers.

59. Paget's disease of the breast is a rare form of ductile carcinoma that is indicated by sores around the nipple. The surrounding skin is often eczematous.

60. Many of the techniques employed in this film also appeared in Popma's instructions. However, some aspects of this film contained an erotic undercurrent. For example, in one image the physician placed his entire hand on the breast and proceeded to rub the breast in his effort to feel "as much of it at one time as possible." Apparently an additional detection method, it seemed inconsistent with earlier recommendations to examine each quadrant of the breast. At another point, after examining the breast, the male doctor followed the narration and checked for lumps in the lymph glands of the neck. While he was doing this, however, he rested his free hand on the naked woman's breast. Finally, the narrator recognized a different, and less endorsed, technique for breast self-examination. "It is believed by some that palpation should also be carried out by the examiner taking a position behind the patient. The examiner's hand is more relaxed in this position. He may be more apt to find a breast mass." A nurse was present throughout the examination, and the narration and image were meant to be instructive. However, I think certain brief moments in this film convey a sexual undercurrent, at least to a contemporary viewer.

61. *Breast Self-Examination*. See also Ross, *Crusade*, 97.

62. *Breast Self-Examination.* The 2:00 P.M. meeting time reflected the shortsightedness of some cancer awareness efforts. Many employed women could not participate in activities or lectures held in the middle of the day.

63. This is a curious addition to the plot because in most films on breast cancer an examination is performed in the film. Eventually, this film too follows that trend, but in a roundabout manner.

64. This dialogue is similar to recent criticism by Susan Love and others that the breast self-examination teaches women to fear their bodies. See Wartic and Felner, "Is Breast Self-Exam Out of Touch?"

65. *Breast Self-Examination.* For excerpts from numerous external reviews of the film, highlighting the *Newsweek* and *Journal of the American Medical Association* reviews as "favorable," see "Breast Self-Examination," 9.

66. "Keep Up with Medicine," 32.

67. "Film Teaches Women to Exam Selves for Cancer," 18.

68. Peggy Lombardo to the author, 1998, in author's possession.

69. Women still accounted for the vast majority of those in attendance; however, the publicity about this viewing in Jacksonville ensured that the topic of breast cancer gained a wider audience.

70. "Breast Self-Examination," 8.

71. Smith, "You Can Escape Breast Cancer," 31.

72. Howard, "How to Prevent 100,000 Cancer Deaths a Year," 41.

73. "Self-Examination for Cancer of the Breast," 84.

74. In the 1950s and 1960s "uterine cancer" was the term frequently used to describe cancer of the cervix, located in the neck of the womb, and to describe uterus cancer, which was located in the body of the womb. Approximately 75 percent of uterine cancers were located in the cervix. In the early 1960s, 14,000 women in the United States died from uterine cancer every year. My discussion follows the usage of these terms in the cancer awareness literature.

75. As this section outlines, Papanicolaou's first effort to introduce screening technology in 1928 attracted little support in the medical world. Throughout the 1950s and 1960s, however, it was championed as an effective cure for cancer. Since the 1970s many critics have challenged its efficacy and accuracy. For a detailed discussion of the history of the Pap smear, see Vayena, "Cancer Detectors."

76. Born in Coumi/Kyme, Greece, in 1883, Papanicolaou earned a doctorate in medicine from the University of Athens in 1904. He then studied in Germany, where he was awarded a Ph.D. in zoology with an emphasis in sex determination. In 1913 he and his wife, Mache Papanicolaou, immigrated to the United States, and he began his career as an assistant in the Department of Pathology at the New York Hospital and assistant in anatomy at Cornell University Medical School. For his earlier cytological research on the estrous cycle of guinea pigs, see Stockard and Papanicolaou, "Existence of a Typical Estrous Cycle in the Guinea Pig."

77. Vayena, "Cancer Detectors," 18–24. In addition to providing vaginal fluid, Mache Papanicolaou worked as an assistant in her husband's lab and supported his research. Vayena also notes that Romanian scientist Aurel Babes

made a simultaneous discovery. Controversy over who deserves credit for the discovery of the vaginal smear still lingers, although most honor Papanicolaou and his Pap smear, except in Romania where it is referred to as the Babes test. Ibid., 22.

78. As Harold Speert has described, "Cancer diagnosis by the cytologic technique, universally known as the Papanicolaou smear, is based on the continuous shedding of cells, like autumn leaves, from all epithelial surfaces." See Speert, *Obstetric and Gynecologic Milestones*, 285. Papanicolaou "examined the vaginal secretion of normal women, and of women known to have histologically proven cancer. He learned the characteristics and the structural variations of the normal exfoliated cells before attempting to study the aberrant traits of the malignant cells. "Exfoliative Cytology," 4.

79. Speert, *Obstetric and Gynecologic Milestones*, 289. Papanicolaou's "first report [in 1928] won no clinical acceptance for the technique, however," Speert writes. "Cytological examination of the vaginal fluid seemed an unnecessary addition to the time-tested diagnostic procedures, endometrial curettage and cervical biopsy."

80. "Exfoliative Cytology," 3.

81. Vayena, "Cancer Detectors," 30. Vayena offers some insightful explanations for the negative response. First, gynecologists were absorbed with other medical issues, such as epithelial cells. Second, practitioners believed in the certainty of the biopsy. Third, surgeons and pathologists wanted to maintain their monopoly on malignant diagnoses.

82. Ibid., 36–44.

83. The vaginal secretion was obtained with the pipette, the secretion was smeared on a small glass slide, and then the slide was fixed and stained for analysis.

84. "Exfoliative Cytology," 4; Papanicolaou and Traut, *Diagnosis of Uterine Cancer by the Vaginal Smear*.

85. Papanicolaou, "Cell Smear Method of Diagnosing Cancer," 202, 203.

86. For examples, see Meigs et al., "Value of Vaginal Smear in the Diagnosis of Uterine Cancer"; and Jones, Neustardter, and Mackenzie, "Value of Vaginal Smears in the Diagnosis of Early Malignancy."

87. Vayena, "Cancer Detectors." Vayena describes the evolution of the Pap smear since 1928 and offers a useful comparison of its application in the Unites States, Britain, and Greece.

88. The continued incidence of cervical cancer in the United States and throughout much of the world, however, has led to a number of criticisms against this technology in recent decades. For examples, see Schroedel and Herndon, "Cervical Cancer Screening Outreach among Low Income, Immigrant, and Minority Communities in Los Angeles County"; Koss, "Papanicolaou Test for Cervical Cancer Detection"; and Jackson, "Screening Method for Cervical Cancer."

89. Many criticisms have been written about this test, especially since the 1970s. Most focus on poor application of the test, its costs, and errors. Nevertheless, it has been a successful screening test to date in the United States. See note 88 for some recent reviews of the test.

90. Papanicolaou, "Cell Smear Method of Diagnosing Cancer," 205.

91. "Doubt on Vaginal Smear," 52.

92. "Exfoliative Cytology," 3.

93. Meigs, *Surgical Treatment of Cancer of the Cervix*. Meigs received his M.D. from Harvard in 1919 and started a career in gynecology. He served as director of gynecology at Vincent Memorial Hospital, Massachusetts General Hospital, and Palmer Memorial Hospital, and by 1942 he was clinical professor of gynecology at Harvard. He specialized in surgical treatment for cervical cancers and frequently served as an ACS spokesperson for female cancers. See Speert, *Obstetric and Gynecologic Milestones*, 401–7.

94. *Time and Two Women*. In the 1970s several feminists groups advocated Pap smear technology for the home. This movement never gained wide support, however.

95. For women comparing popular messages of breast self-examination and vaginal smears, this parallel served to exaggerate the implications of BSE. In BSE a woman detects cancerous lesions, whereas the Pap smear detects precancerous lesions, which can be treated more effectively.

96. Patterson, *Dread Disease*, 137–70.

97. *Cancer Morbidity Series*, 1–10.

98. See also Garcia, "Curability of Carcinoma of the Cervix in the Negro"; Kirchoff and Rigdon, "Frequency of Cancer in the White and Negro"; Christopherson and Parker, "Study of the Relative Frequency of Carcinoma of the Cervix in the Negro."

99. Jones, *Bad Blood*; Reverby, *Tuskegee's Truths*. Reverby's collection of essays by several dozen scholars from a range of disciplines indicates the breadth of scholarly attention that has been directed to this topic since 1972.

100. Hoffman, *Menace of Cancer*, 419.

101. Wright, "Cancer As It Affects the Negro"; Sammons, *Blacks in Science and Medicine*, 329.

102. Mosely, "Cancer and the Negro," 139.

103. The Women's Field Army did extend its work to Harlem, New York, in a deliberate effort to reach African American women. As the New York City Cancer Committee explained, the group was "attempting to accelerate the integration of Negro physicians, technicians, nurses, and medical booth personnel both in municipal and voluntary hospitals." See "Tuberculosis Held Main Harlem Peril."

104. "WOMEN NEED NO LONGER DIE of Their No. 1 Cancer Foe."

105. Christopherson and Parker, "Study of the Relative Frequency of Carcinoma of the Cervix in the Negro," 712–13.

106. "Annual Report 1942–1943 of the Kentucky Division of the Women's Field Army," 7, Filson Historical Society, Louisville, Ky.; "Breast Self-Examination," 7.

107. *Gallup Poll*, 1:495; 2:875, 901, 1138; 3:1926. In 1949, 88 percent of people surveyed believed that a cure for cancer would be found in the next fifty years. In 1965, 77 percent of people surveyed believed a cancer cure would be discovered by 1985.

108. Cartwright, *Screening the Body*, xvii.

109. MacLeod, "Diagnosis: Cancer," 40.
110. The journal that recorded local and national activities of the ACS, *Cancer News*, offered little information about programs designed for African Americans. These programs might have been conducted in local branches that did not send in updates for publication in *Cancer News*.
111. Day, "If the Verdict Is Cancer," 32.

CHAPTER FOUR

1. Scott, *Natural Allies*. See also Skocpol, *Protecting Soldiers and Mothers*; and Skocpol, Munson, Karch, and Camp, "Patriotic Partnerships."
2. *Time Is Life*.
3. At the same time that the ASCC was reorganized into the ACS, the Women's Field Army was renamed the Field Army.
4. Another example of this can be found in the "red door" campaigns of the 1930s, created by Mrs. Ella Rigney, who wanted to encourage women to enter offices to discuss their concerns. Rigney started this project locally, in New York City, in 1938. She hoped to expand it nationally when she joined the Nation Projects Committee of the New York City Cancer Committee. See "Mrs. Rigney in New Cancer Post."
5. The popular description of a complete mastectomy refers to William S. Halsted's radical operation, popularized in 1896 and a common form of breast cancer surgery through the 1970s.
6. Until the 1970s, the majority of breast cancer operations occurred as one-step procedures. A biopsy would be read while the patient remained unconscious. If cancer was found, a surgeon would complete a mastectomy without any further consultation with the patient. A majority of M.D.s believed in this process, although several critics emerged in midcentury. Lerner, *Breast Cancer Wars*, esp. chap. 5.
7. MacLeod, "Diagnosis: Cancer, Recovery: Probable," 40.
8. Ibid.
9. Ibid.
10. Ibid., 136.
11. Kaehele, "I Am Living with Cancer," 123. Kaehele also published a book about her ordeal. Kaehele, *Living with Cancer*.
12. Safford, "Tell Me Doctor," 125.
13. Day, "If the Verdict Is Cancer," 32.
14. Ibid., 43.
15. Ibid.
16. Deutsch and Deutsch, "These 7 People Were Saved from Cancer," 128.
17. "Cancer: On Brink of Breakthroughs," front cover and 103.
18. Ibid., 109.
19. Flexner, "Cancer—I've Had It," 57.
20. F. Cox, "Breast-Pads," U.S. Patent 146,805 (January 27, 1874). The U.S. Patent and Trade Office has issued 228 patents classified as prosthesis/breast (623/7). <www.uspto.gov> (October 3, 2005).

21. Laura Wolfe, "Artificial Breast," U.S. Patent 184,182 (March 6, 1906); Laura Mailleue, "Surgical Breast Substitute," U.S. Patent 1,417,930 (May 20, 1922).
22. Blanche Wiggers, "Breast Adapter," U.S. Patent 2,066,503 (January 5, 1937).
23. Davis, "After Breast Surgery," 129.
24. Yalom, *History of the Breast*, 277.
25. Davis, "After Breast Surgery," 130.
26. Zeiss, "New Life after Breast Cancer," 53.
27. George, "I'm Glad I Had My Breast Removed," 51.
28. Lorde, *Cancer Journals*, 55–77.
29. Although some surgeons adopted conservative surgery early in the twentieth century, until the 1970s the majority of breast cancer surgeries were radical mastectomies. Surgical oncologist Bernard Fisher began challenging the logic of this operation as early as 1966 with his theory of systemic growth. By 1979, Fisher reported long-term studies that concluded no statistical advantage to radical treatment. See Olson, *Bathsheba's Breast*, 129–41.
30. Lasser, "I Had Breast Cancer," 109.
31. "'Cured Cancer Club' Asks 25,000 to Join."
32. References to the Cured Cancer Club appeared occasionally through the 1940s. For examples see "In Cured Cancer Club"; and "Lora Valadon." Valadon was "the first person to qualify for membership in Rhone Island's 'Cured Cancer Club.'"
33. Lasser, *Reach to Recovery*, 10.
34. Ibid., esp. 15.
35. Lasser, "I Had Breast Cancer." Lasser identifies several recovery exercises in this article, including brushing her hair and cleaning.
36. Lasser, *Reach to Recovery*, 20.
37. Ibid., 31.
38. Ibid., 89.
39. *Reach to Recovery Program*. A foreword by Arthur Holleb of the ACS (4–5), an introduction by Terese Lasser (6–9), and descriptions of the Reach to Recovery breast prosthesis (28) provide an overview of the program.
40. *After Mastectomy*. I have been unable to locate production notes for this twenty-one-minute black-and-white film.
41. Although this pamphlet is featured in *After Mastectomy*, I cannot find any copies of it, nor am I sure that it was published for audiences.
42. For an extended discussion of the resonance of the "do not delay" message and its social and cultural underpinnings see Aronowitz, "Do Not Delay."
43. "Pap Test Becoming New Health Habit," 18. For an insightful critique of how the Pap smear gained its status as a powerful screening tool see Casper and Clarke, "Making the Pap Smear into the 'Right Tool' for the Job."
44. See, for example, Schauffler, "Tell Me Doctor."
45. The term "uterine cancer" was used in the 1960s to describe both cancer of the cervix, located in the neck of the womb, and uterus cancer, located in the body of the womb.
46. "Public Education: Uterine Cancer Campaign," 16. See also "Launch Drive to Wipe Out Uterine Cancer."
47. "Cancer: 1961," 13.

48. "Public Education: Conquer Uterine Cancer," 13.
49. Dorothy Height was one of the most effective leaders of the twentieth century. The Schlesinger Library interviewed Height in 1987 and has published this narrative in a bound volume. Her interview reveals a history of familiarity with cancer because her mother nursed cancer patients. See Hill, *Black Women Oral History Project*, vol. 5.
50. Dorothy Height to affiliate presidents, January 3, 1963, Series 10, Box 19, Folder 13, NCNW Collection.
51. Estelle Osbourne to Friends, April 16, 1963, Series 10, Box 19, Folder 13, NCNW Collection.
52. "Pap Test Becoming New Health Habit," 18. See also *Gallup Poll*, vol. 3. Of the 77 percent of women interviewed in 1964 who had heard of/read about the "Pap smear," 48 percent had previously had the examination.
53. *Trends in Cancer*, 12.
54. "Pap Test Becoming New Health Habit," 18.
55. *It's Up to You*.
56. This is a nuanced debate that is still evident today, especially because as more women have mammograms, more cases of ductal carcinoma in situ (DCIS) are treated. Although many cases of DCIS. have been treated aggressively, some scientists argue that the minimal risks associated with the diagnosis do not warrant aggressive treatment. See Tarkan, "Debate on How to Treat Precancerous Breast Disease."
57. *History of Cancer Control*, 1:197–271. See chap. 4, "Detection of Uterine Cervix Cancer."
58. Casper and Clarke, "Making the Pap Smear into the 'Right Tool' for the Job." Vayena's history of the Pap smear adds another dimension to this story. She traces the circumstances that allowed for the transnational exchange of scientific information about cervical screening and the support for clinical trials throughout the United States. Vayena, "Cancer Detectors."
59. Erskine, *Practical X-Ray Treatment*. The second edition was published in 1936, the third in 1947, and the fifth in 1953. Erskine ultimately lost three fingers of his right hand due to radiation overexposure, one testament to the pioneering nature of his work in an era when the debilitating long-term effects of radiation were still unknown. See Clarence B. Luvaas, "Dr. Arthur W. Erskine," obituary article included in "Erskine's 25 Years: Program from Anniversary Celebration," copy owned by Bernice Prunskunas, Cedar Rapids, Iowa. At least one of Erskine's fingers was amputated in April 1937: "Dr. Erskine has had more trouble with the infection in his right ring finger and had it amputated in Akron, Ohio, last week." Erskine to Slye, May 3, 1937, E S193, Erskine Papers, Masonic Grand Lodge Library, Cedar Rapids, Iowa.
60. Kevles offers an insightful examination of the history of radiation in *Naked to the Bone*.
61. Arthur Erskine, "What Can Be Done to Educate the Public to Recognize Cancer of the Breast Earlier?" n.d., E Sp32, Erskine Papers.
62. Interview with Bernice Prunskunas, Cedar Rapids, Iowa, April 29, 1988; "Erskine Helped Point the Way," *Cedar Rapids Gazette*, undated clipping [likely December 1952], in the possession of Prunskunas. Erskine offered

dozens of speeches to women's clubs in the 1930s. See his calendar, E C817, Erskine Papers.

63. Erskine, "X-Ray Treatment of Carcinoma of the Breast," 210. Erskine articulated his concern about women who delayed or refused treatment due to their fear of radical surgery in several papers, including "What Can Be Done to Educate the Public to Recognize Cancer of the Breast Earlier"; and "The Management of Cancer of the Breast," E Sp32a, Erskine Papers.

64. Throughout the 1920s Erskine seemed to support aggressive therapy but wanted the source of the therapy to shift from surgery to radiation. As he wrote in the 1920s, "Realizing the deadliness of the disease, he [the X-ray therapist] must be willing to submit his patients to considerable discomfort, and he must not fear burns, of the skin, or even a few deaths. In order to attain the highest degree of success, and to realize the hopes inspired by recent developments in this art, a certain degree of courage is as essential as a mastery of technical detail." Erskine, "X-Ray Treatment of Carcinoma of the Breast," 211. By the 1930s, his views on aggressive therapy had changed. Erskine responded to patient experience and appeared to have gained greater sensitivity.

65. Erskine, "What Can Be Done to Educate the Public to Recognize Cancer of the Breast Earlier," 6–7.

66. Erskine, "Cancer of the Breast," 1.

67. Erskine, "X-Ray Treatment of Carcinoma of the Breast," 210. Erskine's work with breast cancer challenged conventional surgical treatment, and his work with cervical cancer concentrated on radiation application. As Erskine treated women for cervical cancer, he learned about the pain women associated with cervical cancer treatment. In an effort to respond to these concerns and reduce this pain, Erskine created multiple transvaginal speculums.

68. Erskine, "Curability of Cancer," 1935, p. 3, E Sp32h, Erskine Papers. This speech was located in Erskine's files and contains handwritten notes. However, on the top of the paper is written "Dr. Florence S. Johnston, Convention Federated Women's Clubs, 1935." I do not think Johnston delivered this speech, although it is possible.

69. See Erskine to Mrs. Morden, March 16, 1938, E C817, Erskine Papers. In this letter Erskine asked, "Do speakers usually dress up at meetings of your Women's Club?" Apparently, the talk he was scheduled to give on March 25, 1938, would be one of his first in a woman's club outside Cedar Rapids. Erskine also kept a calendar of his speeches on cancer. Between March 8 and May 5, 1938, various doctors spoke at the Junior League, Clinton Women's Club, Marion Women's Club, the Parent Teacher Association of Lincoln School, St. Wenceslaus Sanctuary Society, the YWCA College Club, and the YWCA "Industrial Girls" Group. See E C817, Erskine Papers.

70. Hennessy to Iowa WFA, January 5, 1938, E W842, Erskine Papers. The Iowa WFA stationery listed the names of its leaders, including Erskine.

71. "Cancer Control," 2, radio talk, Iowa State Medical Society, E Sp32h, Erskine Papers.

72. Erskine, "Cancer Control in Iowa," 2, E Sp32d, Erskine Papers.

73. Ibid.
74. Erskine, "Practical Methods of Reducing the Cancer Death Rate," 17–18, E Sp32d, Erskine Papers. Erskine also questioned how cancer awareness and privatized medicine intersected. In Iowa and other midwestern states, cancer patients without insurance were funneled to one place, the university hospital. Therefore, most medical students, who received their cancer training in university hospitals, treated a disproportionate number of patients with advanced cancers. "This high proportion of advanced cases is apt to give the students the idea that cancer is a hopeless disease," Erskine lamented, "and also fails to teach them the methods of early diagnosis upon which they must later rely." He recognized the influence of economic status in medical care: "Our laws for centralized care of the indigent sick were passed at a time when many students of the cancer problem believed that the ideal procedure would be to treat all cancer patients at no cost to themselves, if necessary, in large, centralized, completely equipped institutions staffed by highly specialized experts in every field of medicine. But experience has shown that such an ideal is difficult to attain. Many people do not like to accept charity. They hate to leave their homes and families and travel long distances to be treated by strangers in unfamiliar surroundings, especially when they fear they may not return alive." Ibid., 14–15.
75. Like many western states, after World War II Iowa established an independent state division of the ACS. Responding to the national interest of the ACS, which urged states to create independent chapters, Iowa incorporated in 1946 "to collect and disseminate information concerning the symptoms, diagnoses, treatment and prevention of cancer, and to aid in cooperation with State and County Medical Societies in the establishment, development, equipment and maintenance of hospitals, clinics, laboratories and other facilities for the treatment and cure of cancer patients, and for research into the cause and cure of cancer." State branches spent at least 60 percent of the money they raised within the state and maintained the authority to develop programs specific to their communities. As one ACS director commented in the early 1950s, "With a great deal of native Iowa pride, we have gone ahead of the national organization on our own in a great many ways." The Iowa chapter won several national awards and recruited support throughout much of the state. Between 1948 and 1951, the number of cancer control meetings in Iowa increased from 800 to 3,033. The Iowa ACS speaker's bureau included 225 doctors, nurses, Iowa division staff, and personnel members who served without pay as educators at these meetings. In 1951 the Iowa ACS chapter received the national ACS "tops in the nation" recognition for programs in education, service, and research. Dr. Cornelius Rhoads, the director of the New York Memorial Hospital, stated, "The Iowa division has the best program of research and education of any ACS division I have yet seen." Moreover, it raised more money per capita than any other ACS chapter. The 1951 annual fund drive collected $521,664 (as compared to its first drive in 1947 that raised $253,000). "Report By Your Executive Director," 1951, 1, E Am35ir, Erskine Papers.
76. Ibid., 1, 3–5. Zimmerer suggested, "We have been cautious in predicting the

saving of lives even though we have concrete evidence that some women as a result of seeing this film sought prompt medical advice and were subjected to surgery." "The Twenty-First Semi-Annual Report," 1, E C16, Erskine Papers.

77. Erskine to Sinclair, July 13, 1948, E Am35ie, Erskine Papers; Drs. Willis E. Brown, J. T. Bradbury, and O. F. Kraushaar, "The Papanicolaou Test in the Cancer Control Program," n.d. [though data suggests 1945], E P197, Erskine Papers.

78. Naomi Doebel, "C.R. to Be First Iowa City to Use New Cancer Test," *Gazette*, October 16, 1948, clipping in E P197, Erskine Papers; Brown, Bradbury, and Kraushaar, "Papanicolaou Test in the Cancer Control Program." I cannot ascertain if the women volunteered for this test, if it was presented as routine, or if any coercion was involved.

79. Erskine to Dr. Morgan, September 8, 1947, E Am35ie, Erskine Papers. At least three cytologists in Cedar Rapids were trained to read the smears, one of whom was trained specifically for this purpose in Boston by Dr. Joseph Meigs.

80. Doebel, "C.R. to Be First Iowa City to Use New Cancer Test."

81. Erskine to Dr. Morgan, October 30, 1948, E P197, Erskine Papers; Doebel, "C.R. to Be First Iowa City to Use New Cancer Test."

82. Erskine to Sinclair, July 13, 1948, E Am35ie, Erskine Papers.

83. "Report By Your Executive Director," 1951, 6, E Am35ir, Erskine Papers.

84. *Cancer: A Manual For the Public*, prepared and distributed by the Cancer Committee of the Iowa State Medical Society, the Iowa Division of the Field Army of the American Cancer Society, and the Division of Cancer Control of the State Department of Health, undated [probably 1951], p. 25, E P96a, Erskine Papers.

85. Ibid., 38.

86. Erskine, "Cancer of the Breast," 2.

87. Ibid.

88. Lerner, *Breast Cancer Wars*, chap. 5. Lerner has traced the medical debates about the best treatment for breast cancer. Specifically, in the 1950s those studying biological data doubted the influence of aggressive surgery. As Lerner writes, "These critics, many of whom lived outside of the United States, conducted sophisticated statistical analyses that challenged the standard assumptions that early detection of breast cancer was indeed 'early' and that radical surgery actually 'cured' breast cancer patients." Ibid., 92.

CHAPTER FIVE

1. Both Betty Ford and Happy Rockefeller announced their breast cancer diagnoses in 1974.

2. A mammography demonstration project was planned in 1971, the National Cancer Institute joined it in 1972, and women enrolled in the Breast Cancer Detection Demonstration Project in 1973. Beginning in 1976, public criticism of radiation's risks caused a reevaluation of the project. See Lerner, *Breast Cancer Wars*, 206–22.

3. In 1978 Ann Marcou and Mimi Kaplan founded Y-ME National Breast Cancer Organization "to provide support to fellow breast cancer patients and their loved ones." Ann Marcou to the author, November 7, 2003.

4. Ehrenreich, "Welcome to Cancerland," 45.

5. Betty Ford had earned a reputation as a feminist. She supported the Equal Rights Amendment, as well as women's reproductive rights. It is not surprising that she used her personal diagnosis to direct publicity to breast cancer.

6. "News Conference," Box 3, Folder "O," Document H3, BFP.

7. Olson, *Bathsheba's Breast*, 125–27.

8. "Speech for Commonwealth Awards," 98-NLF-042 Files, "T & E, 1998," BFP.

9. Krueger, "Death Be Not Proud."

10. Lerner, *Breast Cancer Wars*, 208–9.

11. For examples, see Kushner, *Breast Cancer*; and Rollins, *First You Cry*.

12. The Health Insurance Program of New York funded the first randomized trial of mammography under the direction of statistician Sam Shapiro and radiologist Philip Strax in 1963. By 1966 Strax had reported that screening led to earlier detection of breast cancer. See Lerner, *Breast Cancer Wars*, 197–203.

13. Experiments in radiology that suggested that X-ray could indicate early stages of breast cancer began as early as 1913. See Lerner, *Breast Cancer Wars*, 111.

14. Gershon-Cohen, "Chest Cradle for Roentgen Examination of Female Breast."

15. *History of Cancer Control*, 1:273–318.

16. Ibid., 1:285–95.

17. Spicer, "New Weapons against Breast Cancer," 48.

18. See Lerner, *Breast Cancer Wars*, 196–222. Lerner traces the controversy and confusion over the benefits of mammography. John C. Bailer III, a statistician for the National Cancer Institute and the deputy associate director for cancer control, wrote a 1976 critique that questioned the value of mammography and its risk. Subsequently, journalists challenged the ACS at its annual meeting, and investigative work continued to expose the potential and actual errors with the trial through 1977.

19. Ratcliff, "Facts about Breast Cancer," 68.

20. Lescher, "Painless New Way to Detect Breast Cancer," 13.

21. "Better Way," 159, 160.

22. Lerner, "Philip Strax."

23. *History of Cancer Control*, esp. 1:295–302.

24. Thermography was a screening device based on heat sensors and blood flow. This was ineffective and ultimately abandoned.

25. "Breast Cancer," in *1975 Cancer Facts and Figures* (New York: ACS, 1976), in Weidenfeld Social Files, Box 2, "9/27/74 breast surgery," BFP. See also *History of Cancer Control*, 1:297–300.

26. *ACS Annual Report*, 1973, 4.

27. Lerner, *Breast Cancer Wars*, 246.

28. Connell, "Detecting Breast Cancer," 40.

29. Ibid., 40.
30. Ibid., 42.
31. Olson, *Bathsheba's Breast*, 208–11; Lerner, *Breast Cancer Wars*, 209–13.
32. Brody, "Radiation Benefits, Risks in Breast Cancer Debated"; Greenberg, "X-Ray Mammography." For additional analysis of this controversy, see Olson, *Bathsheba's Breast*; and Lerner, *Breast Cancer Wars*.
33. Greenberg, "X-Ray Mammography," 739.
34. Olson, *Bathsheba's Breast*, 211.
35. The "high risk" designation was so general, however, that it included a large percentage of the female population. Lerner, *Breast Cancer Wars*, 215–22.
36. Bernard Fisher was one of the most notable surgeons who had challenged conventional (Halsted radical) surgery since 1958. By 1974, he and other physicians had published numerous articles that indicated that radical surgery offered no additional benefits to conservative surgery in most cases of breast cancer. For example, see Fisher, "Surgical Dilemma."
37. Kushner, *Breast Cancer*, 3–31.
38. Shirley Temple Black and Rosamond Campion made a similar point in 1972 when each insisted on a two-stage mastectomy. Blakeslee, "Shirley Temple Black Makes Plea Again"; and Klemesrud, "New Voice in Debate on Breast Surgery."
39. Lerner, *Breast Cancer Wars*, 115–40.
40. Ibid., 170.
41. Kushner, *Breast Cancer*.
42. "For Immediate Release," September 28, 1974, 1, 3, "O'Neill Files, General Health," Box 3, BFP.
43. See Lerner, *Breast Cancer Wars*, chap. 8, for an extensive analysis of the transformation in breast cancer treatment and feminists' responses to it.
44. "For Immediate Release, the White House Press Conference of Dr. William Lukash," September 28, 1974, O'Neill Files, General, "Health" 10, Box 3, BFP; Morgen, *Into Our Own Hands*.
45. Letter to Betty Ford, October 1974, White House Subject Files and Social Files (hereinafter WHSFSF), FL 13-8 "11/1/74–11/7/74," Box 25, BFP.
46. Bix, "Disease Chasing Money and Power"; BWHC, *Our Bodies, Ourselves*.
47. "For Immediate Release," September 28, 1974, 3. Fouty was reluctant to embrace moderate and conservative shifts in surgery and shared these opinions with the Fords. They agreed to follow his advice and have a complete mastectomy as needed.
48. "9/27/74 breast surgery (1)," Weidenfeld Files, Box 2, BFP.
49. Telegrams and letters to Ford, "PP 10-2-1 8/9/74–10/4/74," Subject File, Box 42, BFP.
50. The President Gerald R. Ford Library kept 10 percent of the letters. I only found one letter that criticized Ford's decision to make her diagnosis public. The Betty Ford archivist, Leesa Tobin, told me that the sample was representative and, indeed, few complained about Ford's public discussion of breast cancer.
51. Letter to Betty Ford, May 15, 1975, "FL 13 1/29/75–6/27/75," Boxes 24–25, WHSFSF, BFP.

52. Letter to Betty Ford, January 28, 1975, "FL 13 1/29/75–6/27/75," Boxes 24–25, WHSFSF, BFP.
53. Letter to Betty Ford, January 15, 1975, "FL 13 1/16/75–1/27/75," Box 26, WHS-FSF, BFP.
54. Letter to Betty Ford, March 5, 1975, "FL 13 1/29/75–6/27/75," Boxes 24–25, WHSFSF, BFP.
55. Letter to Betty Ford, April 14, 1975, "FL 13 1/29/75–6/27/75," Boxes 24–25, WHSFSF, BFP.
56. Letter to Betty Ford, November 24, 1974, "FL 13-8 11/8/74–11/30/74," Boxes 24–25, WHSFSF, BFP.
57. Letter to Betty Ford, January 1975, "FL 13-8 1/28/75–1/31/75," Box 26, WHS-FSF, BFP.
58. Letter to Betty Ford, January 8, 1975, "FL 13-8 1/28/75–1/31/75," Box 26, WHSFSF, BFP.
59. DR #6 (WHSF-BM), "Get well messages—Betty Ford's Cancer Surgery," BFP.
60. Letter to Betty Ford, October 1, 1974, "FL 13-8 10/1/74–10/21/74," Boxes 24–25, WHSFSF, BFP.
61. Letter to Betty Ford, September 27, 1974, "FL 13-8 10/1/74–10/21/74," Boxes 24–25, WHSFSF, BFP.
62. Letter to Betty Ford, October 11, 1974, "FL 13-8 11/8/74–11/30/74," Boxes 24–25, WHSFSF, BFP.
63. Letter to Betty Ford, not dated, "FL 13-8 11/8/74–11/30/74," Box 25, WHS-FSF, BFP.
64. Letter to Betty Ford, November 9, 1974, "FL 13-8, 1/8/75–1/15/75," Box 25, WHSFSF, BFP.
65. Letter to Gerald Ford, October 31, 1974, "FL 13-8 10/1/74–10/21/74," Boxes 24–25, WHSFSF, BFP.
66. Letter to Betty Ford, October 9, 1974, "FL 13-8 11/1/74–11/7/74," Boxes 24–25, WHSFSF, BFP.
67. "Press Questions of Governor Nelson A. Rockefeller," 1, November 24, 1974. Rockefeller Family Archives, RG 26, Press Files Series, Box 23, "Articles, Mrs. Nelson A. Rockefeller."
68. Ibid., 2.
69. "In Case It Should Happen to You," 11. Rockefeller Family Archives, RG 26, Press Files Series, Box 23, "Articles, Mrs. Nelson A. Rockefeller."
70. Maisel, "How You Can Double Your Chances against Cancer," 90.
71. Lerner, *Breast Cancer Wars*, 81.
72. Olson, *Bathsheba's Breast*, 90–91.
73. Lerner, *Breast Cancer Wars*, 104–5. As Lerner notes, Crile stopped performing Halsted mastectomies in 1955, "likely becoming the only surgeon in the United States to have done so." Ibid., 104. Fisher headed the National Surgical Adjuvant Breast and Bowel Project and began collecting data for a scientific comparison of different treatment options. Ibid., 137–38. North Americans John L. Madden, Hugh Auchincloss, and Henry Leis were also critics of radical surgery in the United States in the 1950s. Barney Crile's reports in

the early 1960s about his success with conservative surgery also challenged the notion of radical surgery, as did Vera Peters's work in Canada. By the late 1960s, hostile medical debates emerged, as well as the call for randomized controlled trials. Barron Lerner offers an excellent overview of this era in *Breast Cancer Wars*, chaps. 5–6.

74. Women who requested modified surgeries often enraged physicians who dismissed their opinions. As one example, see Ruzek, *Women's Health Movement*, 114.

75. On "patients in revolt," see Lerner, *Breast Cancer Wars*, chap. 7. See also Altman, *Waking Up, Fighting Back*, 171–72; and Kushner, *Alternatives*, chap. 11.

76. Nolen, "Operation Women Fear Most," 52.

77. Ibid.

78. Ibid.

79. Ibid., 56.

80. *Breast Cancer: Where We Are.*

81. Xerography is a "process for copying graphic matter by the action of light on an electrically charged photoconductive insulating surface in which the latent image is developed with resinous powder." *Merriam-Webster Dictionary* <http://www.m-w.com> (August 26, 2005).

82. See More and Millian, *Empathic Practitioner.*

83. Evans, *Born for Liberty*, 289.

84. BWHC, *Our Bodies, Our Selves*, 12.

85. Marieskind and Ehrenreich, "Toward Socialist Medicine," 38.

86. Ruzek, *Women's Health Movement*, 26.

87. Ibid., 53.

88. "'Pap' by Mail," 59.

89. BWHC, *Our Bodies, Our Selves*, 1.

90. Ruzek, *Women's Health Movement*, esp. chap. 3.

91. BWHC, *Our Bodies, Our Selves*, 1.

92. BWHC, *Our Bodies, Ourselves*, 263.

93. Ibid., 265.

94. BWHC, *Our Bodies, Ourselves*, 2d ed., 127.

95. Ibid., 148.

96. Ibid., esp. 130–35.

97. "Preface," <www.ourbodiesourselves.org/about/1973obos.asp> (October 8, 2005).

98. "Mammogram Debate."

99. Brody, "Choosing to Have Annual Mammograms."

100. As two examples, the Susan G. Komen Breast Cancer Foundation (established in 1982) and the National Alliance of Breast Cancer Coalitions (established in 1986) were formed to educate women, advocate for women, and ensure funding for breast cancer research.

101. See "Physicians and Patients Neglect Ovarian Cancer," 277.

102. "Edith's Christmas Story," *All in the Family*, December 22, 1973, viewed at the Museum of Radio and Television, New York, N.Y.

1. The National Alliance of Breast Cancer Coalitions began in 1986 for educational and informational resources and to support patient advocacy; the Susan G. Komen Breast Cancer Foundation started in 1982 in memory of founder Nancy Brinker's sister; the National Breast Cancer Coalition was founded in 1991 and is the country's largest breast cancer advocacy group today.
2. Since 1970, numerous women have challenged the medical profession and its response to breast cancer. I highlight the work of a few women here as a mere sampling of some of the major concerns that have been articulated in recent decades. Historian Barron Lerner has written an excellent account of the feminist response to medical controversies in *Breast Cancer Wars*; see esp. chaps. 7–8.
3. Kushner, *Breast Cancer*.
4. Lorde, *Cancer Journals*.
5. Ehrenreich, "Welcome to Cancerland," 52.
6. "Cult or Culture?" 5.
7. ACS, "Estimated New Cancer Cases and Deaths by Sex." Although some statistical studies note a decline in breast cancer mortality since the 1990s, others challenge this claim due to the increase of cancer in situ detection and its classification.
8. Amy Sue Bix offers a good comparison of the activism in AIDS and breast cancer awareness in "Diseases Chasing Money and Power."
9. National Breast Cancer Coalition, "History, Goals, and Accomplishments," <http://www.natlbcc.org> (January 15, 2005).
10. This decline is most evident in industrialized countries. However, the Pap smear has not eradicated cervical cancer. See Schroedel and Herndon, "Cervical Cancer Screening Outreach among Low Income, Immigrant, and Minority Communities in Los Angeles County."
11. Phillips, "Pit Bulls, Children Unsafe Combination."
12. Love, "Detecting Breast Cancer before It Starts"; Wartic and Felner, "Is the Breast Self-Exam Out of Touch?"
13. Clow, *Negotiating Disease*, xiii.

Bibliography

ARCHIVAL SOURCES

Ann Arbor, Michigan
President Gerald R. Ford Library
  Betty Ford Papers

Baltimore, Maryland
Alan Mason Chesney Medical Archives, Johns Hopkins University
  Joseph Colt Bloodgood Papers
  William Halsted Papers

Cedar Rapids, Iowa
Masonic Grand Lodge Library
  Arthur W. Erskine Papers

Chicago, Illinois
American Medical Association Archives
  Historic Health Fraud Collection

College Park, Maryland
National Archives and Records Administration
  Motion Picture, Sound, and Video Collection

Louisville, Kentucky
Filson Historical Society
  Annual Report 1942–1943 of the Kentucky Division of the Women's
      Field Army

New York, New York
Columbia University
  Oral History Research Collection
    Mary Lasker Oral History Project
  Rare Book and Manuscript Library
    Mary Lasker Papers
Museum of Radio and Television
  July 27, 1950, *The Quick and the Dead*, part 4
  January 27, 1952, *Ed Murrow on Cancer*
  May 2, 1959, *Tactic* (World premiere of a program designed to find
      ways in which America's great creative people can help with the
      fight of cancer. Cast included Alfred Hitchcock.)

December 22, 1973, *All in the Family*
March 31, 1974, *CBS segment on Laetrile*
November 11, 1974, *Medical Center: Tainted Lady*
February 26, 1979, *ABC news segment on Sheila Stainback re: mastectomy*
   and surgical reconstruction
June 16, 1980, *Choosing Suicide*
September 27, 1981, *60 Minutes segment on fraud cancer clinic*
March 15, 1983, *St. Elsewhere*
1990, *Why, Charlie Brown, Why*
April 1990, *NPR's Susan Stamberg interviews Nina Hyde re: breast cancer*
March 28, 1992, *Beverly Hills on breast cancer*
September 14, 1993, *ABC News Special: The Other Epidemic: What Every*
   Woman Needs to Know about Breast Cancer
1994, *Spanish Cancer Assn. ad on breast cancer*
November 15, 1994, *NYPD Blue*
Winter 1994, *Dyke TV on breast cancer*
February 6, 1995, *Chicago Hope on breast cancer*
Young Women's Christian Association
   Health Collection

North Tarrytown, New York
Rockefeller Archive Center
   Record Group 26, Nelson A. Rockefeller, Vice Presidential

Washington, D.C.
American Association of University Women Archives
   Cancer Files
   General Federation of Women's Clubs Correspondence
General Federation of Women's Clubs
   Marjorie Illig Papers
   Grace Morrison Poole Papers
Library of Congress Manuscript Division
   Florence Deakins Becker Papers
Library of Congress Prints and Photographs Division
   American Cancer Society. *Atencion: Viva mas!* [1965–1980]. Call no. POS
      6—U.S., no. 994.
   Corra la voz acera de los Mamogramas. Washington, D.C.: National Institutes
      of Health, 1999.
Mary McLeod Bethune House
   National Council of Negro Women Collection

FILMS

After Mastectomy. American Cancer Society, Oregon Division, 1958. 21 minutes.
   A drama of one woman's rehabilitation after mastectomy and a discussion of
   her fears and concerns. Viewed at Library of Congress, Film Division.
Breast Cancer: Where We Are. Made by Stan Lang, Inc., presented by the American
   Cancer Society, 1973. Directed and photographed by Michael Zingale; writ-

ten by Mal Marquith and Gerald Prueitt; executive producer Donald S. Hillman; associate producer Mary Ensign; edited by Edgar A. Fricke, Sr.; sound by Al Mian and Michael Tromer. Viewed at Library of Congress, Film Division.

Breast Self-Examination: A Film For Women's Groups on Breast Cancer. American Cancer Society, National Cancer Institute, U.S. Public Health Service, 1950. 15.5 minutes. Film demonstrates the breast self-examination. Viewed at Library of Congress, Film Division.

Cancer: The Problem of Early Diagnosis. American Cancer Society and U.S. National Cancer Institute, 1949. 32 minutes. Viewed at Library of Congress, Film Division.

Cancer (Virus). National Educational Television Film Service, 1960.

Choose to Live. American Society for the Control of Cancer in cooperation with the U.S. Public Health Service, and produced by the U.S. Department of Agriculture, Extension Service, 1940. Directed by W. Allen Luey; medical director C. V. Akin, M.D.; script by Clifton Read; production manager Ernest Bryan; and photographer Carl Turvey. 18 minutes. Viewed at the National Archives and Record Administration, Film Division; see Record Groups 90.1.1 and 90.1.2.

The Great Peril. New York: American Society for the Control of Cancer, 1920. 15 minutes.

Inside Magoo. American Cancer Society, 1960. 14.5 minutes.

It's Up to You. American Cancer Society, 1970. 13 minutes. This film follows a woman to a lecture on uterine cancer. The lecture and, consequently, the film stress the importance of annual Pap smears. Viewed at Library of Congress, Film Division.

Journey into Darkness. Made by Trio Productions, American Cancer Society, 1969. Film warns viewers about the dangers of quacks and the value of a reputable physician when dealing with cancer.

Life Saving Fingers. American Cancer Society, Idaho Division, 1948. 21 minutes. Viewed at Library of Congress, Film Division.

Living Insurance. Written by Stanford L. Sobel and directed by Leo Seltzer; produced by Sturgis-Grant Productions; sponsored by the American Cancer Society, Idaho Division; medical direction by Raymond L. White, M.D.; technical assistance, Alfred M. Popma, M.D., and Mrs. Grant Hess, 1953. Follows a thirty-four-year-old man during an annual examination that offers "living insurance" against cancer. Viewed at Library of Congress, Film Division.

Luisa Tenia Razon. Produced by Juan E. Viguie Jr., made by Viguie Film Production, 1968. 11 minutes. Spanish-language film that explores a woman's concerns about uterine cancer and the advice of her daughter-in-law.

Man Alive. Written by Bill Scott and William S. Roberts; produced by Stephen Bosustow; directed by William T. Hurtz; animation by Philip Monroe, Cecil Surry, and Rudy Larriva; music by Benjamin Lees; and voice by Victor Perrin. Produced by United Productions of America. Sponsored by the American Cancer Society, and distributed by Heartland Area Education Agency, 1952. 11 minutes. Animated film that compares a man's car troubles to his case of indigestion, which may also be an early warning of cancer, emphasizing the seven warning signs of cancer and the importance of early detection. Viewed at Library of Congress, Film Division.

The Odyssey of Dr. Pap. Narrated by E. G. Marshall and made by Harry Olesker Productions, American Cancer Society, 1969. 30 minutes. Film traces the career of Dr. Papanicolaou, beginning with his career in Greece. Film stresses the importance of annual Pap smears for women.

Psychological Aspects of the Nurse-Patient Relationship in Cancer. American Cancer Society, 1969. 22 minutes. Film teaches nurses how to deal with the complicated emotional reactions of recently diagnosed cancer patients.

Recovery after Mastectomy. New York American Cancer Society, 1970. Film depicts a patient's experience after mastectomy. A nurse and a volunteer visit and demonstrate exercises and prosthesis options.

Sappy Homiens. American Cancer Society, 1956. Viewed at Library of Congress, Film Division.

Time and Two Women. Written by Joseph Meigs; distributed by American Cancer Society, 1957. 20 minutes. The American Cancer Society sent the author a copy of this film that follows the cases of two women with uterine cancer.

Time Is Life. Directed by Francis Thompson; camera by Peter Glushanok; produced by the American Cancer Society and Farm Film Foundation, 1946. 19 minutes. This black-and-white film emphasizes the importance of early detection through the narrative of one woman's experience with breast cancer.

The Traitor Within. American Cancer Society, John Sutherland Productions; directed by George Gordon and story by Norm Wright; animation by Pete Burness, Irven Spence, Elmer Swanson; art direction by Bernice Polifka and music by Paul Smith, 1946. 10 minutes. Animated cartoon compares normal cells and cancer cells. Film emphasizes the importance of early detection. Viewed at Library of Congress, Film Division.

Wide Wide World: The Creative Spirit. Executive producer, Barry Wood; produced by Gerald Green; directed by Dick Schneider; written by Lou Salaman; and music composed and conducted by David Broekman. NBC Kinescope, 1957. Viewed at Library of Congress, Film Division.

The Winners: Checkups for Life. American Cancer Society Production, produced by Audio Productions Film, 1968. 8 minutes. This film, directed primarily at men, stresses the importance of regular examinations.

PRIMARY AND SECONDARY TEXTS

"11,600 Cancer Cases Aided by Group Here." *New York Times*, October 28, 1932.

"16,000 Women." *Cancer News*, Winter 1957, 2–9.

"25,000 Hear Cancer Talk." *Washington Post*, January 2, 1923.

"Abby Aldrich Rockefeller, 1874–1948." Rockefeller Archive Center. <http://archive.rockefeller.edu/bio/abby>. December 10, 2004.

Adams, Diane L., ed. *Health Issues for Women of Color.* Thousand Oaks, Calif.: Sage, 1995.

Adams, Samuel Hopkins. *The Health Master*. New York: Houghton Mifflin Company, 1913.

———. "What Can We Do about Cancer?" *Ladies' Home Journal*, May 1913, 21–22.

"Alfred Marion Popma, M.D., F.A.C.R." *Idaho Statesman*, August 30, 1996.

Altman, Roberta. *Waking Up, Fighting Back: The Politics of Breast Cancer*. Boston: Little, Brown and Company, 1996.

American Cancer Society. "Annual ACS Report." *Cancer News*. 1947–.

———. *ACS Annual Report, 1973*. New York: American Cancer Society, 1974.

———. *Cancer News*. 1947–.

———. "Estimated New Cancer Cases and Deaths by Sex for All Sites, US, 2004." <http://www.cancer.org/downloads/MED/page4.pdf>. December 15, 2004.

———. *Reach to Recovery Manual*. New York: American Cancer Society, 1972.

American College of Surgeons Commission on Cancer 75th Anniversary Commemorative Booklet: 1922–1997. Chicago: American College of Surgeons, 1997.

American Society for the Control of Cancer. *The American Society for the Control of Cancer: Its Objects and Methods and Some of the Visible Results of Its Work*. New York: American Society for the Control of Cancer, 1925.

———. *The ASCC: Report for the Year Ended March 31, 1928*. New York: American Society for the Control of Cancer, 1928.

———. *Bulletin of the American Society for the Control of Cancer*. 1914–20.

———. *Cancer and the Public Health*. New York: American Society for the Control of Cancer, 1916.

———. *Cancer Control: Report of an International Symposium Held under the Auspices of the American Society for the Control of Cancer*. Chicago: Surgical Publishing Company, 1927.

———. *Certificate of Incorporation of the American Society for the Control of Cancer, Incorporated*. New York: ASCC, 1922.

———. *Facts about Cancer*. New York: American Society for the Control of Cancer, 1914.

———. *History of the American Society for the Control of Cancer: 1913–1943*. New York: American Society for the Control of Cancer, 1944.

———. *Important Facts for Women about Tumors*. New York: American Society for the Control of Cancer, 1931.

———. *There Shall Be Light!* New York: American Society for the Control of Cancer, 1936.

———. *Women's Field Army: Organized to Save Human Life*. New York: American Society for the Control of Cancer, 1937.

Angier, Natalie. "Confronting Cancer: Getting Used to Life, Long Life, with Cancer." *New York Times*, April 9, 2002.

Apple, Rima D. "Constructing Mothers: Scientific Motherhood in the Nineteenth and Twentieth Centuries." *Social History of Medicine* 8 (1995): 161–78.

———. *Mothers and Motherhood: Readings in American History*. Columbus: Ohio State University Press, 1997.

——, ed. *Women, Health, and Medicine in America: A Historical Handbook*. New York: Garland Publishers, 1990.

Aronowitz, Robert A. "Do Not Delay: Breast Cancer and Time, 1900–1970." *Milbank Quarterly* 79 (2001): 355–86.

"Attack on Cancer Likened to War." *New York Times*, March 5, 1939.

Austoker, Joan. *A History of the Imperial Cancer Research Fund, 1902–1986*. Oxford, U.K.: Oxford University Press, 1988.

Baker, Rachel. *The First Woman Doctor: The Story of Elizabeth Blackwell*. New York: Julian Messner, 1944.

Barney, Sandra Lee. *Authorized to Heal: Gender, Class, and the Transformation of Medicine in Appalachia*. Chapel Hill: University of North Carolina Press, 2000.

Batt, Sharon. *Patient No More: The Politics of Breast Cancer*. Charlottetown, Canada: Gynergy Books, 1994.

Bazell, Robert. *Her 2: The Making of Herceptin, a Revolutionary Treatment for Breast Cancer*. New York: Random House, 1998.

Beard, Mary Ritter. *Woman as Force in History: A Study in Traditions and Realities*. New York: Macmillan, 1946.

——. *Woman's Work in Municipalities*. New York: D. Appleton and Company, 1915.

Bell, E. Moberly. *Storming the Citadel: The Rise of the Woman Doctor*. London: Constable, 1953.

Berney, Adrienne. "Streamlining Breasts: The Exaltation of Form and Disguise of Foundation in 1930s' Ideals." *Journal of Design History* 14 (2001): 327–42.

Bernstein, Nancy R. *The First One Hundred Years: Essays on the History of the American Public Health Association*. Washington, D.C.: American Public Health Association, 1972.

"The Better Way." *Good Housekeeping*, May 1963, 159–61.

Bix, Amy Sue. "Disease Chasing Money and Power: Breast Cancer and AIDS Activism Challenging Authority." *Journal of Policy History* 9 (1997): 5–32.

"Bi-Yearly Cancer Examinations." *Medical Woman's Journal*, May 1942, 151.

Blakeslee, Sandra. "Shirley Temple Black Makes Plea Again; Tells Women to Avoid Delay in Breast Cancer Check." *New York Times*, November 9, 1972.

Bland, P. Brooke. "Cancer in Women." *Hygeia*, May 1930, 460.

Bloodgood, Edith Holt, and Victor H. Long, eds. *Index to the Writings of Joseph Colt Bloodgood, M.D.* Baltimore: Lord Baltimore Press, 1936.

Bloodgood, Joseph Colt. "Cancer of the Cervix: The Immediate Necessity for Earlier Diagnosis and Treatment." *American Journal of Cancer* 16 (September 1932): 1238–45.

——. "Cancer Prevention—A Task in Education." *Journal of the American Association of University Women* 25 (June 1932): 219–22.

——. "The Evidence of Value of Education in Cancer Control." In ASCC, *Cancer Control: Report of an International Symposium Held under the Auspices of the American Society for the Control of Cancer*, 163–64. Chicago: Surgical Publishing Company, 1927.

——. "The Greatest Scourge in the World." *Good Housekeeping*, February 1929, 59, 196–206.

————. "What Everyone Should Know about Cancer." *Scientific American*, April 10, 1915, 231.

Boston Women's Health Collective. *Our Bodies, Our Selves: A Course by and for Women*. Boston: New England Free Press, 1971.

————. *Our Bodies, Ourselves: A Book by and for Women*. New York: Simon and Schuster, 1973.

————. *Our Bodies, Ourselves: A Book by and for Women*. 2d ed. New York: Simon and Schuster, 1976.

Boyd, Peggy. *The Silent Wound: A Startling Report on Breast Cancer and Sexuality*. Reading, Mass.: Addison-Wesley Publishers, 1984.

Boylan, Anne. *The Origins of Women's Activism*. Chapel Hill: University of North Carolina Press, 2002.

Bradley, Mary Hastings. *Pattern of Three*. New York: D. Appleton-Century Company, 1937.

Brandt, Alan. *No Magic Bullet: Social History of Venereal Disease in the United States*. New York: Oxford University Press, 1985.

"Breast Self-Examination: A Courageous New Stride in Public Health Education." *Cancer News* 4 (October 1950): 3–9.

Brody, Jane. "Choosing to Have Annual Mammograms." *New York Times*, February 5, 2002.

————. "Radiation Benefits, Risks in Breast Cancer Debated." *New York Times*, March 28, 1976.

Bud, R. F. "Strategy in American Cancer Research after World War II: A Case Study." *Social Studies of Science* 8 (1978): 425–59.

Bynum, W. F., and Roy Porter, eds. *Companion Encyclopedia of the History of Medicine*. 2 vols. New York: Routledge, 1993.

Calatayud, Jesús, and Ángel González. "History of the Development and Evolution of Local Anesthesia Since the Coca Leaf." *Anesthesiology* 98 (June 2003): 1503–8.

Cameron, Virginia. *Tuberculosis Medical Research: National Tuberculosis Association, 1904–1955*. New York: National Tuberculosis Association, 1959.

"The Campaign against Cancer." *Journal of the Iowa State Medical Society* 27 (March 1937): 117.

"The Campaign against Cancer—Educational, Experimental, and Clinical." *Scientific American*, May 11, 1912, 428.

Campbell, William Francis. "The Early Recognition of Carcinoma Mammae." *Transactions of the Associated Physicians of Long Island* 1 (June 1898): 124–32.

Campion, Rosamond. *The Invisible Worm*. New York: Macmillan, 1972.

"Cancer: 1961, Uterine Program Winning Support of Women's Clubs." *Cancer News* 15 (1961): 13.

"Cancer and the Meat Eater." *Current Literature* 43 (November 1907): 560.

"Cancer and the Negro." *Opportunity* 15 (February 1937): 51–53.

"Cancer Campaign Planned." *New York Times*, September 12, 1921.

"Cancer Education Via Radio." *American Journal of Public Health* 26 (June 1936): 644–45.

Cancer: Facts Which Every Adult Should Know. Washington, D.C.: U.S. Public Health Service, 1919.

"Cancer Fund Drive Is Started in City." *New York Times*, October 31, 1934.

"Cancer Group Opens Booths for Recruits." *New York Times*, March 24, 1937.

Cancer Information Clearinghouse. *Breast Cancer: Annotated Bibliography of Public, Patient, and Professional Information and Educational Materials.* Bethesda, Md.: Department of Health, Education, and Welfare, 1979.

"Cancer Is Treated Like This." *Good Housekeeping*, May 1940, 44–45, 96.

Cancer Morbidity Series. Washington, D.C.: U.S. Public Health Service, 1950–52.

"Cancer: On Brink of Breakthroughs." *Life Magazine*, May 5, 1958, 102–12.

Cantor, David. "Cancer." In *Companion Encyclopedia of the History of Medicine*, edited by W. F. Bynum and Roy Porter, 1:537–60. New York: Routledge, 1993.

———. "The MRC's Support for Experimental Radiology During the Inter-War Years." In *Historical Perspectives on the Role of the MRC: Essays in the History of the Medical Research Council of the United Kingdom and Its Predecessor, the Medical Research Committee, 1913–1953*, edited by Joan Austoker and Linda Bryder, 181–204. Oxford, U.K.: Oxford University Press, 1989.

Carmichael, Erskine. *The Pap Smear: Life of George N. Papanicolaou.* Springfield, Ill.: Charles C. Thomas Publisher, 1973.

Carnett, J. B. "Cancer of the Breast." *Hygeia*, March 1930, 261–62.

Cartwright, Lisa. *Screening the Body: Tracing Medicine's Visual Culture.* Minneapolis: University of Minnesota Press, 1995.

Casper, Monica J., and Adele E. Clarke. "Making the Pap Smear into the 'Right Tool' for the Job: Cervical Cancer Screening in the USA circa 1940–1945." *Social Studies of Science* 28 (April 1998): 255–90.

"Celebrity Fete Tonight." *New York Times*, January 9, 1936.

"Charity Event Today at the Biltmore." *New York Times*, June 5, 1935.

"Cheatle Endorses Three Cancer Aids." *New York Times*, October 10, 1931.

Christopherson, William, and James Parker. "A Study of the Relative Frequency of Carcinoma of the Cervix in the Negro." *Cancer* 13 (July/August 1960): 711–13.

Cianfrani, Theodore. *A Short History of Obstetrics and Gynecology.* Springfield, Ill.: Charles C. Thomas Publisher, 1960.

"Cleveland Cancer Medal Awarded." *Medical Woman's Journal*, October 1942, 305.

Clow, Barbara. *Negotiating Disease: Power and Cancer Care, 1900–1950.* Montreal: McGill–Queen's University Press, 2001.

———. "Who's Afraid of Susan Sontag? Or, The Myths and Metaphors of Cancer Reconsidered." *Social History of Medicine* 14 (2001): 293–312.

Coe, Henry C. "Address of the President." *Transactions of the American Gynecological Society* 38 (1913): 3–21.

Connell, Elizabeth B. "Detecting Breast Cancer." *Redbook*, July 1973, 40, 42.

"The Control of Cancer." *Outlook* 104 (August 16, 1913): 840.

Cott, Nancy F. *The Bonds of Womanhood: "Woman's Sphere" in New England, 1780–1835.* New Haven, Conn.: Yale University Press, 1977.

———. *The Grounding of Modern Feminism.* New Haven, Conn.: Yale University Press, 1987.

Cowan, Ruth Schwartz. *A Social History of American Technology.* New York: Oxford University Press, 1997.

Creager, Angela N. H., Elizabeth Lunbeck, and Londa Schiebinger, eds. *Feminism* in *Twentieth-Century Science, Technology, and Medicine*. Chicago: University of Chicago Press, 2001.

Crile, George. *A Biological Consideration of the Treatment of Breast Cancer*. Springfield, Ill.: Charles C. Thomas, 1967.

————. "Management of Breast Cancer: Limited Mastectomy." *International Journal of Radiation Oncology, Biology, Physics* 2 (1977): 969–73.

————. "Results of Conservative Operations for Breast Cancer." *Archives of Surgery* 120 (1985): 746–51.

————. "Results of Simple Mastectomy without Irradiation in the Treatment of Operative Stage I Cancer of the Breast." *Annals of Surgery* 168 (1968): 330–36.

————. "Results of Simplified Treatment of Breast Cancer." *Surgery, Gynecology, and Obstetrics* 118 (1964): 517–23.

————. "Surgery in the Days of Controversy." *Journal of the American Medical Association* 262 (1989): 258.

Crile, George, C. B. Esselstyn, R. E. Hermann, et al. "Partial Mastectomy for Carcinoma of the Breast." *Surgery, Gynecology, and Obstetrics* 136 (1973): 929–33.

Crook, Marion. *My Body: Women Speak Out about Their Health Care*. New York: Plenum Press, 1995.

"Cult or Culture?" *Harper's Magazine* 304 (February 2002): 4–5, 85.

"'Cured Cancer Club' Asks 25,000 to Join." *New York Times*, March 25, 1938.

"Curing Cancer by the Finsen Phototherapy System." *Current Literature* 27 (March 1900): 230.

Dally, Ann. *Women under the Knife: A History of Surgery*. New York: Routledge, 1991.

Dan, Alice J., ed. *Reframing Women's Health: Multidisciplinary Research and Practice*. Thousand Oaks, Calif.: Sage, 1994.

Davis, Loyal. *Fellowship of Surgeons: A History of the American College of Surgeons*. Chicago: American College of Surgeons, 1988.

Davis, Maxine. "After Breast Surgery." *Good Housekeeping*, September 1954, 28.

Day, Emerson. "If the Verdict Is Cancer." *Woman's Home Companion*, January 1955, 32–33, 43, 46.

Demaitre, Luke. "Medieval Notions of Cancer: Malignancy and Metaphor." *Bulletin of the History of Medicine* 72 (1998): 609–37.

De Moulin, Daniel. *A History of Surgery: With Emphasis on the Netherlands*. Boston: Martinus Nijhoff Publishers, 1988.

————. *A Short History of Breast Cancer*. Boston: Martinus Nijhoff Publishers, 1983.

Deutsch, Patricia, and Ron Deutsch. "These 7 People Were Saved from Cancer." *Ladies' Home Journal*, March 1957, 128–29, 231–32.

"Dinner to Aid Education." *New York Times*, January 6, 1936.

"Doubt on Vaginal Smear." *Newsweek*, November 17, 1947, 52.

Dow, Karen Hassey. *Contemporary Issues in Breast Cancer*. Sudbury, Mass.: Jones and Bartlett, 1996.

"Dr. Hoffman Dies, Actuarial Expert." *New York Times*, February 25, 1946, 20.

Dreifus, Claudia, ed. *Seizing Our Bodies: The Politics of Women's Health*. New York: Vintage Books, 1978.

Duffy, John. *From Humors to Medical Science: A History of American Medicine.* Urbana: University of Illinois Press, 1993.

———. *The Healers: The Rise of the Medical Establishment.* New York: McGraw-Hill, 1976.

"Easier Steps Are the Best First Steps." *American Journal of Public Health* 24 (August 1934): 899.

"Edith Nourse Rogers, 1881–1960." <http://bioguide.congress.gov>. December 2004.

Ehrenreich, Barbara. "Welcome to Cancerland: A Mammogram Leads to a Cult of Pink Kitsch." *Harper's Magazine* 303 (November 2001): 43–53.

Ehrenreich, Barbara, and Deirdre English. *Complaints and Disorders: The Sexual Politics of Sickness.* Old Westbury, N.Y.: Feminist Press, 1973.

———. *For Her Own Good: 150 Years of the Experts' Advice to Women.* New York: Doubleday, 1978.

Elston, Mary Ann. "Reclaiming Our Bodies: Health Handbooks by and for Women." *Women's Studies International Quarterly* 2 (1979): 117–25.

Encyclopaedia Britannica Online. <http://search.eb.com>. August 26, 2005.

Epstein, Julia. *The Iron Pen.* Madison: University of Wisconsin Press, 1989.

———. "Writing the Unspeakable: Fanny Burney's Mastectomy and the Fictive Body." *Representations* 16 (Autumn 1986): 131–66.

Erskine, Arthur Wright. "Cancer of the Breast." *Wisconsin Medical Journal,* September 1935, 1–2.

———. *Practical X-Ray Treatment.* St. Paul, Minn.: Bruce Publishing Company, 1931.

———. "X-Ray Treatment of Carcinoma of the Breast." *Illinois Medical Journal,* March 1922, 209–11.

Evans, Sarah M. *Born for Liberty: A History of Women in America.* New York: Free Press Paperbacks, 1997.

"Exfoliative Cytology." *Cancer News* 2 (June 1948): 3–11.

"Facing Cancer with Courage." *Hygeia,* May 1931, 421–23.

"Fighting Cancer." *Science News Letter* 33 (February 5, 1938): 83–85.

"Film Teaches Women to Exam Selves for Cancer." *Science News Letter* 58 (July 8, 1950): 18.

Fisher, Bernard. "The Surgical Dilemma in the Primary Therapy of Invasive Breast Cancer: A Critical Appraisal." *Current Problems in Surgery* 7 (1970): 3–53.

Fisher, Bernard, and Marc Gebhardt. "A Commentary on the Role of the Surgeon in Primary Breast Cancer." *Breast Cancer Research and Treatment* 1 (1986): 17–26.

———. "The Evolution of Breast Cancer Surgery: Past, Present, and Future." *Seminars in Oncology* 5 (December 1978): 385–94.

Flexner, Marion W. "Cancer—I've Had It." *Ladies' Home Journal,* May 1947, 57, 150.

Foner, Eric, ed. *The New American History.* Philadelphia: Temple University Press, 1990.

Ford, Betty, with Chris Chase. *Betty, A Glad Awakening.* New York: Doubleday Press, 1987.

————. *Times of My Life*. New York: Harper and Row, 1978.

Gallup Poll: Public Opinion, 1935–1971. 3 vols. New York: Random House, 1972.

Garcia, Manuel. "The Curability of Carcinoma of the Cervix in the Negro." *Southern Medical Journal* 45 (February 1952): 145–50.

Gardner, Kirsten E. "From Cotton to Silicone: Breast Prosthesis before 1950." In *Artificial Parts, Practical Lives: Modern History of Prosthetics*, edited by Katherine Ott, David Serlin, and Stephen Mihm, 102–19. New York: New York University Press, 2002.

————. "Hiding the Scars: A History of Post-Mastectomy Breast Prostheses, 1945–2000." *Enterprise and Society* 1 (September 2000): 565–90.

Garraty, John A., and Marc C. Carnes, eds. *American National Biography*. Vol. 10. New York: Oxford University Press, 1999.

Garrett, Laurie. *The Coming Plague: Newly Emerging Diseases in a World Out of Balance*. New York: Farrar, Straus and Giroux, 1994.

Garrison, Fielding H. *An Introduction to the History of Medicine*. Philadelphia: W. B. Saunders Company, 1914.

George, Charlotte. "I'm Glad I Had My Breast Removed." *Today's Health*, August 1957, 50–51.

Gershon-Cohen, Jacob. "Chest Cradle for Roentgen Examination of Female Breast." *Radiology* 28 (1937): 234–36.

Gilman, Charlotte Perkins. *The Yellow Wallpaper*. New York: Feminist Press, 1973.

Gimlin, Debra L. *Body Work: Beauty and Self-Image in American Culture*. Berkeley: University of California Press, 2002.

Grady, Denise. "In Breast Cancer Data, Hope, Fear, and Confusion." *New York Times*, January 26, 1999.

Greenberg, Daniel. "X-Ray Mammography—Background to a Decision." *New England Journal of Medicine* 295 (September 23, 1976): 739–40.

Haller, John S. *American Medicine in Transition, 1840–1910*. Urbana: University of Illinois Press, 1981.

Halsted, William S. "The Results of Operations for the Cure of Cancer of the Breast Performed at the Johns Hopkins Hospital from June, 1889 to January, 1894." *Annals of Surgery* 20 (1894): 497–555.

————. "The Results of Radical Operations for the Cure of Carcinoma of the Breast." *Annals of Surgery* 46 (1907): 1–19.

Handley, W. Sampson. *Cancer of the Breast and Its Operative Treatment*. London: John Murray, 1906.

Hartnagel, Arthur C. "Cancer of the Cervix." Senior thesis, 1925.

Hellman, Geoffrey. "Mary Roberts Rinehart: For 35 years She Has Been America's Best-Selling Lady Author." *Life*, February 25, 1946, 55–56.

Higginbotham, Evelyn Brooks. *Righteous Discontent: The Women's Movement in the Black Baptist Church, 1880–1920*. Cambridge, Mass.: Harvard University Press, 1993.

Hill, Ruth Edmonds, ed. *The Black Women Oral History Project*. Vol. 5. Westport, Conn.: Meckler, 1991.

Hirshberg, Leonard Keene. "How Cancer May Be Prevented." *Harper's Weekly*, March 1913, 11.

A History of Cancer Control in the United States, 1946–1971. 4 vols. Bethesda, Md.: Department of Health, Education, and Welfare, 1977.

Hoffman, Frederick L. *Cancer and Civilization.* Newark, N.J.: Prudential Press, 1923.

———. *Cancer in the Native Races.* Newark, N.J.: Prudential Press, 1926.

———. *Cancer Increase and Overnutrition.* Newark, N.J.: Prudential Press, 1927.

———. *The Menace of Cancer.* Newark, N.J.: Prudential Press, 1913.

———. *The Mortality of Cancer throughout the World.* Newark, N.J.: Prudential Press, 1915.

———. *On the Causation of Cancer: An Address Delivered before the American Association for Cancer Research.* Newark, N.J.: Prudential Press, 1924.

———. *Some Cancer Facts and Fallacies.* Newark, N.J.: Prudential Press, 1925.

———. *Some Essential Statistics of Cancer Mortality throughout the World.* New York: American Medical Association, 1915.

———. *Some Final Results of the San Francisco Cancer Survey.* Newark, N.J.: Prudential Press, 1929.

Holmes, Jane. "I Didn't Have Cancer." *Woman's Home Companion,* June 1948, 12.

"Homer Truett Bone, 1883–1970." <http:// bioguide.congress.gov>. January 10, 2005.

Howard, Clive. "How to Prevent 100,000 Cancer Deaths a Year." *Woman's Home Companion,* September 1950, 40–41, 126–27.

Hufnagel, Vicki, with Susan K. Golant. *No More Hysterectomies.* New York: Penguin Books, 1989.

Hufnagel, Vicki, and Robert Pokras. *Hysterectomies in the United States, 1965–84.* In *Vital and Health Statistics,* Series 13, No. 92. Washington, D.C.: Government Printing Office, 1987.

Hummel, Sherilyn J., and Marie Lindquist. *If It Runs in Your Family: Ovarian and Uterine Cancer, Reducing Your Risk.* New York: Bantam Books, 1992.

Hunt, Nancy. *A Colonial Lexicon of Birth Ritual, Medicalization, and Mobility in the Congo.* Durham, N.C.: Duke University Press, 1999.

Hushberg, Leonard Keene. "How Cancer May Be Prevented." *Harper's Weekly,* March 29, 1913, 11.

"I'm Not Afraid of Cancer." *Hygeia,* February 1938, 138–40, 174.

"The Importance of Cancer Education." *Hygeia,* March 1933, 234–35.

"In Cured Cancer Club." *New York Times,* August 9, 1946.

The India Office List for 1932. London: Harrison and Sons, 1933.

Jackson, Nancy Beth. "Screening Method for Cervical Cancer." *New York Times,* March 16, 1999.

James, Arthur G. *Cancer Prognosis Manual.* New York: American Cancer Society, 1966.

Johnson, Edwin. *Breast Cancer, Black Woman.* Montgomery, Ala.: Van Slyke and Bray, 1993.

Jones, C. A., T. Neustardter, and L. L. Mackenzie. "The Value of Vaginal Smears in the Diagnosis of Early Malignancy." *American Journal of Obstetrics and Gynecology* 49 (February 1945): 15.

Jones, James. *Bad Blood: The Tuskegee Syphilis Experiment.* New York: Free Press, 1981.

Kaehele, Edna. "I Am Living with Cancer." *Woman's Home Companion*, September 1952, 30–31, 122–23, 140–48.

———. *Living with Cancer*. New York: Doubleday, 1952.

Kaiser, Jocelyn. "Army Doles Out First $210 million." *Science* 266 (October 14, 1994): 212.

Keenan, Kevin L. "Albert Davis Lasker." American National Biography Online, <http://www.anb.org>. February 1, 2000.

"Keep Up with Medicine." *Good Housekeeping*, November 1955, 32.

Kennedy, Samuel. *Samuel Hopkins Adams and the Business of Writing*. Syracuse, N.Y.: Syracuse University Press, 1999.

Kent, Rosemary May. "An Evaluation of the Health Education Program of the American Cancer Society, North Carolina Division." M.S. thesis, University of North Carolina at Chapel Hill, 1949.

Kerber, Linda. "Separate Spheres, Female Worlds, Woman's Place: The Rhetoric of Women's History." *Journal of American History* 75 (June 1988): 9–39.

Kevles, Bettyann Holtzmann. *Naked to the Bone: Medical Imaging in the Twentieth Century*. New Brunswick, N.J.: Rutgers University Press, 1997.

Kirchoff, Helen, and R. H. Rigdon. "Frequency of Cancer in the White and Negro." *Southern Medical Journal* 49 (August 1956): 834–41.

Kirschner, Don S. *The Paradox of Professionalism: Reform and Public Service in Urban America, 1900–1940*. New York: Greenwood Press, 1986.

Klemesrud, Judy. "New Voice in Debate on Breast Surgery." *New York Times*, December 12, 1972.

Kolata, Gina. "Vying for the Breast Vote." *New York Times*, November 3, 1996.

Koss, Leopald. "The Papanicolaou Test for Cervical Cancer Detection: A Triumph and a Tragedy." *Acta Cytologica* 34 (September 1990): 607.

Krementsov, Nikolai. *The Cure: A Story of Cancer and Politics from the Annals of the Cold War*. Chicago: University of Chicago Press, 2002.

Krueger, Gretchen Marie. "Death Be Not Proud: Children, Families, and Cancer in Postwar America." *Bulletin of the History of Medicine* 78 (Winter 2004): 836–63.

Kushner, Rose. *Alternatives: New Developments in the War on Breast Cancer*. Cambridge, Mass.: Kensington Press, 1984.

———. *Breast Cancer: A Personal History and Investigative Report*. New York: Harcourt Brace Jovanovich, 1975.

"Lack of Light as a Prevalent Cause of Cancer." *Current Opinion*, April 1914, 285.

Lasser, Terese. "I Had Breast Cancer." *Coronet*, April 1954, 109–12.

———. *Reach to Recovery: A Manual for Women Who Have Had Radical Breast Surgery*. New York: Reach to Recovery Foundation, 1953.

Lasser, Terese, and William Kendall Clarke. *Reach to Recovery*. New York: Simon and Schuster, 1972.

"Launch Drive to Wipe Out Uterine Cancer." *Today's Health*, September 1961, 69.

Lawrence, Christopher, ed. *Medical Theory, Surgical Practice: Studies in the History of Surgery*. London: Routledge, 1992.

Leavitt, Judith Walzer. *The Healthiest City: Milwaukee and the Politics of Health Reform*. Princeton, N.J.: Princeton University Press, 1982.

———. *Typhoid Mary: Captive to the Public's Health*. Boston: Beacon Press, 1996.

————, ed. *Women and Health in America*. Madison: University of Wisconsin Press, 1984.

Leavitt, Judith Walker, and Ronald L. Numbers, eds. *Sickness and Health in America: Readings in the History of Medicine and Public Health*. Madison: University of Wisconsin Press, 1978.

Leopold, Ellen. *A Darker Ribbon: Breast Cancer, Women, and Their Doctors in the Twentieth Century*. Boston: Beacon Press, 1999.

Lerner, Barron H. *The Breast Cancer Wars: Hope, Fear, and the Pursuit of a Cure in Twentieth-Century America*. New York: Oxford University Press, 2001.

————. "Fighting the War on Breast Cancer: Debates over Early Detection, 1945 to the Present." *Annals of Internal Medicine* 129 (July 1, 1998): 74–78.

Lescher, Ruth. "Painless New Way to Detect Breast Cancer." *Ladies' Home Journal*, April 1963, 13, 18, 146.

Levine, Susan. *Degrees of Equality: The American Association of University Women and the Challenge of Twentieth-Century Feminism*. Philadelphia: Temple University Press, 1995.

Liebstein, A. M. "The Rational and Prophylactic Treatment of Cancer." *National Eclectic Medical Association Quarterly* 33 (March 1942): 1–8.

Lipkin, Hilda C., ed. *Index to the Annals of Medical History, 1917–1942*. New York: Harry Schuman, 1946.

Little, C. C. *Cancer: A Study for Laymen*. New York: American Society for the Control of Cancer, 1944.

Lockwood, C. B. *Cancer of the Breast: An Experience of a Series of Operations and Their Results*. London: Oxford University Press, 1913.

"Lora Valadon." *New York Times*, September 16, 1946.

Lorde, Audre. *The Cancer Journals*. Argyle, N.Y.: Spinsters Ink, 1980.

Love, Susan. "Detecting Breast Cancer before It Starts." *New York Times*, October 7, 2002.

Love, Susan M., with Karen Lindsey. *Dr. Susan Love's Breast Book*. Reading, Mass.: Addison-Wesley, 1990.

MacLeod, Lily. "Diagnosis: Cancer, Recovery: Probable." *Ladies' Home Journal*, January 1951, 40–41, 132–34, 136.

Maisel, Albert Q. "How You Can Double Your Chances against Cancer." *Woman's Home Companion*, January 1954, 40–41, 80, 89–91.

Major, Ralph H. *A History of Medicine*. Springfield, Ill.: Charles C. Thomas, 1954.

"The Mammogram Debate: Highlights of Recent Research and Recommendations." *Washington Post*, February 5, 2002.

Marcus, Alan I. *Cancer from Beef: DES, Federal Food Regulation, and Consumer Confidence*. Baltimore: Johns Hopkins University Press, 1994.

Marieskind, Helen I., and Barbara Ehrenreich. "Toward Socialist Medicine: The Women's Health Movement." *Social Policy* 6 (1975): 34–42.

Marshino, Ora. "Breast Cancer." *Hygeia*, March 1945, 176–77, 201–2.

Martin, Emily. *The Woman in the Body: A Cultural Analysis of Reproduction*. Boston: Beacon Press, 1987.

Maulitz, Russell C. "Rudolf Virchow, Julius Cohnheim and the Program of Pathology." *Bulletin of the History of Medicine* 52 (1978): 162–82.

McGregor, Deborah Kuhn. *From Midwives to Medicine: The Birth of American Gynecology*. New Brunswick, N.J.: Rutgers University Press, 1998.

———. *Sexual Surgery and the Origins of Gynecology*. New York: Garland Publishing, 1989.

Mead, Kate Campbell. *Medical Women of America: A Short History of the Pioneer Medical Women of America and a Few of Their Colleagues in England*. New York: Froben Press, 1933.

Medvei, Victor Cornelius. *A History of Endocrinology*. Lancaster, Mass.: MTP Press Limited, 1982.

Meigs, Joseph Vincent. *Surgical Treatment of Cancer of the Cervix*. New York: Grune and Stratton, 1954.

Meigs, J. V., R. M. Graham, M. Fremont-Smith, I. Kapnick, and R. W. Rawson. "The Value of Vaginal Smear in the Diagnosis of Uterine Cancer." *Surgery, Gynecology, and Obstetrics* 77 (November 1943): 449.

Meyerowitz, Joanne. *Not June Cleaver: Women and Gender in Postwar America, 1945–1960*. Philadelphia: Temple University Press, 1994.

Morantz, Regina Markell. "The Perils of Feminist History." *Journal of Interdisciplinary History* 4 (1974): 649–60.

Morantz, Regina Markell, Cynthia Stodola Pomerleau, and Carol Hansen Fenichel. *In Her Own Words: Oral Histories of Women Physicians*. Westport, Conn.: Greenwood Press, 1982.

More, Ellen Singer, and Maureen Millian. *The Empathic Practitioner: Empathy, Gender, and Medicine*. New Brunswick, N.J.: Rutgers University Press, 1994.

Morgen, Sandra. *Into Our Own Hands: The Women's Health Movement in the United States: 1969–1980*. New Brunswick, N.J.: Rutgers University Press, 2002.

Morrow, Albert Sidney. *Cancer: A Manual for High School Teachers*. New York: New York City Cancer Committee, 1944.

Moseley, James E. "Cancer and the Negro." *Crisis* 56 (May 1949): 138–39, 156.

Moss, Ralph W. *The Cancer Industry: Unraveling the Politics*. 1980; New York: Paragon, 1989.

"Mrs. C. P. Huntington's Gift." *New York Times*, May 24, 1902.

"Mrs. Rigney in New Cancer Post." *New York Times*, December 18, 1944.

"Mrs. S. A. Clark, 69, Welfare Worker." *New York Times*, January 13, 1949.

Mulhearn, Christine. "Women in Philanthropy: Mrs. Russell Sage (Margaret Olivia Slocum), 1828–1918." Cambridge, Mass.: Kennedy School of Government Case Program no. 1565.0, 2000.

Narrigan, Deborah. "My-Pap: The Do-It-Yourself Pap Smear." *The Network News*, November 1, 1991.

National Breast Cancer Coalition: "A Grassroots Advocacy Effort." [This is undated and conversations with the National Breast Cancer Coalition suggest it was published in 1993.]

Nechas, Eileen, and Denise Foley. *Unequal Treatment: What You Don't Know about How Women Are Mistreated by the Medical Community*. New York: Simon and Schuster, 1994.

"Negro Health Week to Begin April 5." *New York Times*, February 15, 1925.

"New Basis Urged for War on Cancer." *New York Times*, March 26, 1938.

"A New Director Elected." *Woman's Medical Journal*, December 1943, 304.

Nolen, William A. "The Operation Women Fear Most." *McCall's*, April 1971, 52, 54, 56.

Nuland, Sherwin B. *Doctors: The Biography of Medicine*. New York: Vintage Books, 1988.

Oakley, Ann. *Essays on Women, Medicine, and Health*. Edinburgh: Edinburgh University Press, 1993.

O'Dowd, Michael, and Elliot E. Philipp. *The History of Obstetrics and Gynaecology*. New York: Parthenon Publishing Group, 1994.

Olson, James S. *Bathsheba's Breast: Women, Cancer, and History*. Baltimore: Johns Hopkins University Press, 2002.

——. *The History of Cancer: An Annotated Bibliography*. New York: Greenwood Press, 1989.

Orenstein, Peggy. "Scheduling Breast Cancer in Prime Time." *New York Times*, September 28, 1997.

Ott, Katherine. *Fevered Lives: Tuberculosis in American Culture since 1870*. Cambridge, Mass.: Harvard University Press, 1996.

Palmer, Gretta. "I Had Cancer." *Ladies' Home Journal*, July 1947, 143–48, 150, 152–53.

"'Pap' by Mail." *Newsweek*, February 4, 1963, 59–60.

"Pap Smear." *Encyclopaedia Britannica Online*, <http://search.eb.com>. December 2004.

"Pap Test Becoming New Health Habit." *Cancer News* 18 (Spring 1964): 18.

Papanicolaou, George. "The Cell Smear Method of Diagnosing Cancer." *American Journal of Public Health* 38 (February 1948): 202–5.

Papanicolaou, George, and Herbert F. Traut. *Diagnosis of Uterine Cancer by the Vaginal Smear*. Cambridge, Mass.: Harvard University Press Commonwealth Fund, 1943.

Park, Roswell. "The Campaign against Cancer." *American Review of Reviews* 48 (December 1913): 712.

Patterson, James T. *The Dread Disease: Cancer and Modern American Culture*. Cambridge, Mass.: Harvard University Press, 1987.

Peitzman, Steven J. *A New and Untried Course: Woman's Medical College and Medical College of Pennsylvania, 1850–1998*. New Brunswick, N.J.: Rutgers University Press, 2000.

Phillips, Jeanne. "Pit Bulls, Children Unsafe Combination." *Cincinnati Enquirer*, June 28, 2004.

"Physicians and Patients Neglect Ovarian Cancer." *Science News Letter* 85 (May 1964): 277.

Plotkin, David. "And Bad News about Breast Cancer." *Atlantic Monthly*, June 1996, 53–82.

Porter, Dorothy. "Public Health." In *Companion Encyclopedia of the History of Medicine*, edited by W. F. Bynum and Roy Porter, 1231–61. New York: Routledge, 1993.

"Post-War Control of Cancer Is Urged." *New York Times*, October 15, 1943.

"Prevention and Cure of Cancer." *Independent*, July 3, 1916, 34.

Proctor, Robert. *Cancer Wars: How Politics Shapes What We Know and Don't Know about Cancer*. New York: Basic Books, 1995.

———. *The Nazi War on Cancer*. Princeton, N.J.: Princeton University Press, 1999.

"Progress Hailed in Cancer Clubs." *New York Times*, April 14, 1940.

"Public Education: Conquer Uterine Cancer." In American Cancer Society, "Annual ACS Report [1963]," *Cancer News* 17 (1963): 13.

"Public Education: Uterine Cancer Campaign." In American Cancer Society, "Annual ACS Report [1961]," *Cancer News* 16 (1962): 16.

Ratcliff, J. D. "Facts about Breast Cancer." *Reader's Digest*, March 1963, 68.

Ratcliff, Kathryn Strother, ed. *Healing Technology: Feminist Perspectives*. Ann Arbor: University of Michigan Press, 1989.

Rather, L. J. *The Genesis of Cancer: A Study in the History of Ideas*. Baltimore: Johns Hopkins University Press, 1978.

———. "Johannes Müller, Theodor Schwann, Matthias Schleiden, Jacob Henle, and the Nature of Plant and Animal Cells." In *Johannes Müller and the Nineteenth-Century Origins of Tumor Cell Theory*, by L. J. Rather, Patricia Rather, and John B. Frerichs, 1–55. Canton, Mass.: Science History Publications, 1986.

Reach to Recovery Program. New York: American Cancer Society, 1974.

Reagan, Leslie. "Engendering the Dread Disease: Women, Men, and Cancer." *American Journal of Public Health* 87 (1998): 1779–87.

Records of the National Association of Colored Women's Clubs, 1895–1992. Microfilm. Bethesda, Md.: University Publications of America, 1993–.

"Relation of Beer to Cancer." *Current Literature*, September 1903, 347.

"Report of the Committee on the Ways and Means in the Matter of Impressing Physicians and Educating the Public in the Necessity of Early Diagnosis and Operation in Cancer." *Transactions of the American Gynecological Society*, 1913, 462–63.

"Report of the Surgeon General of the U.S. Army to the Secretary of War, 1931." In *Annual Report of the Surgeon General of the Army: 1928–1931*. Washington, D.C.: Government Printing Office, 1931.

Rettig, Richard A. *Cancer Crusade: The Story of the National Cancer Act of 1971*. Princeton, N.J.: Princeton University Press, 1977.

Reverby, Susan, ed. *Tuskegee's Truths: Rethinking the Tuskegee Syphilis Study*. Chapel Hill: University of North Carolina Press, 2000.

Reverby, Susan, and David Rosner, eds. *Health Care in America: Essays in Social History*. Philadelphia: Temple University Press, 1979.

"Rich Women Begin a War on Cancer." *New York Times*, April 23, 1913.

Richards, Evelleen. *Vitamin C and Cancer: Medicine or Politics*. London: Macmillan, 1991.

Rigney, Ella Hoffman. *A History of the American Society for the Control of Cancer: 1913–1947*. New York: American Society for the Control of Cancer, n.d. [ca. 1947].

Risse, Guenter B., Ronald L. Numbers, and Judith Walzer Leavitt. *Medicine Without Doctors: Home Health Care in American History*. New York: Science History Publications, 1977.

Rollins, Betty. *First You Cry*. Philadelphia: Lippincott, 1976.

Rosen, George. *The History of Miners' Diseases: A Medical and Social Interpretation*. New York: Schuman's, 1942.

———. *A History of Public Health*. New York: MD Publications, 1958.

———. *The Specialization of Medicine*. New York: Froben Press, 1944.

Rosenberg, Charles. *The Care of Strangers: The Rise of America's Hospital System*. New York: Basic Books, 1987.

———. *Explaining Epidemics and Other Studies in the History of Medicine*. New York: Cambridge University Press, 1992.

———. *Healing and History: Essays for George Rosen*. New York: Science History Publications, 1979.

———. *No Other Gods: On Science and American Social Thought*. Baltimore: Johns Hopkins University Press, 1997.

Ross, Ishbel. *Child of Destiny: The Life Story of the First Woman Doctor*. New York: Harper, 1949.

Ross, Walter. *Crusade: The Official History of the American Cancer Society*. New York: Arbor House, 1987.

Rosser, Sue V. *Women's Health—Missing from U.S. Medicine*. Bloomington: Indiana University Press, 1994.

Rupp, Leila J. *Worlds of Women: The Making of an International Women's Movement*. Princeton, N.J.: Princeton University Press, 1997.

Ruzek, Sheryl Burt. *The Women's Health Movement: Feminist Alternatives to Medical Control*. New York: Praeger, 1978.

———. *Women's Health: Complexities and Differences*. Columbus: Ohio State University Press, 1997.

Safford, Henry B. "Tell Me Doctor." *Ladies' Home Journal*, December 1953, 39, 124–25.

Saleeby, C. W. *The Conquest of Cancer*. New York: Frederick A. Stokes Company, 1907.

Sammons, Vivian Ovelton. *Blacks in Science and Medicine*. New York: Hemisphere Publishing Company, 1990.

Schauffler, Goodrich C. "Tell Me Doctor." *Ladies' Home Journal*, February 1962, 28.

Schroedel, Jean R., and Brooke Herndon. "Cervical Cancer Screening Outreach among Low Income, Immigrant, and Minority Communities in Los Angeles County." *International Journal of Public Administration* 27 (2004): 83–108.

Scott, Anne Firor. *Natural Allies: Women's Associations in American History*. Urbana: University of Illinois Press, 1991.

Scott, Joan. "Gender: A Useful Category for Historic Analysis." *American Historical Review* 91 (December 1986): 1053–75.

Schwartz, Samuel M., Donald W. Slater, Fred P. Heydrick, and Gillian R. Woollett. "AIBS News: A Report of the AIBS Peer-Review Process for the US Army's 1994 Breast Cancer Initiative." *Bioscience* 45 (1995): 558.

"Self-Examination for Cancer of the Breast." *Ladies' Home Journal*, August 1952, 84.

Shaughnessy, Donald F. "The Story of the American Cancer Society." Ph.D. diss., Columbia University, 1957.

Shryock, Richard H. *The Development of Modern Medicine: An Interpretation of the Social and Scientific Factors Involved.* Philadelphia: University of Pennsylvania Press, 1936.

——. "The Historian Looks at Medicine." *Bulletin of the Institute of the History of Medicine* 5 (December 1937): 887–94.

——. *Medicine and Society in America, 1660–1860.* New York: New York University Press, 1960.

——. *Medicine in America: Historical Essays.* Baltimore: Johns Hopkins University Press, 1966.

——. *National Tuberculosis Association, 1904–1954: A Study of the Voluntary Health Movement in the United States.* 1957; New York: Arno Press, 1977.

——. "Women in American Medicine." *Journal of the American Medical Women's Association* 5 (1950): 371–79.

Skocpol, Theda. *Protecting Soldiers and Mothers: The Political Origins of Social Policy in the United States.* Cambridge, Mass.: Belknap Press, 1992.

Skocpol, Theda, Ziad Munson, Andrew Karch, and Bayliss Camp. "Patriotic Partnerships: Why Great Wars Nourished American Civic Volunteerism." In *Shaped by Way and Trade: International Influences on American Political Identity,* edited by Ira Katznelson and Martin Shefter, 134–80. Princeton, N.J.: Princeton University Press, 2001.

Sigerist, Henry E. *American Medicine.* New York: W. W. Norton, 1934.

——. *On the History of Medicine.* New York: MD Publications, 1960.

Singer, Charles. *A Short History of Medicine: Introducing Medical Principles to Students and Non-Medical Readers.* New York: Oxford University Press, 1928.

Smith, C. H. "You Can Escape Breast Cancer." *Hygeia,* January 1950, 30–31.

Smith, Susan. *Sick and Tired of Being Sick and Tired: Black Women's Health Activism in America, 1890–1950.* Philadelphia: University of Pennsylvania Press, 1995.

Smith-Rosenberg, Carroll. "The Female World of Love and Ritual: Relations between Women in Nineteenth-Century America." *Signs* 1 (Autumn 1975): 1–29.

"Some Results of National Cancer Week." *American Journal of Public Health* 13 (April 23, 1922): 296–99.

Sontag, Susan. *Illness as Metaphor.* Harmondsworth: Penguin, 1978.

Speert, Harold. *Obstetric and Gynecologic Milestones: Essays in Eponymy.* New York: Macmillan, 1958.

Spicer, Betty Coe. "New Weapons against Breast Cancer." *Ladies' Home Journal,* June 1962, 48.

"Spread of Cancer Greatest in Men." *New York Times,* March 8, 1931.

Stabiner, Karen. *To Dance with the Devil: The New War on Breast Cancer.* New York: Delacorte Press, 1997.

Stanton, Annette L., and Sheryle J. Gallant. *The Psychology of Women's Health: Progress and Challenges in Research and Application.* Washington, D.C.: American Psychological Association, 1995.

Starr, Paul. *The Social Transformation of American Medicine.* New York: Basic Books, 1982.

Stern, Phyllis Noerager. *Women, Health, and Culture.* Washington, D.C.: Hemisphere Publishing Company, 1986.

Stevens, Barbara. *Not Just One in Eight*. Deerfield Beach, Fla.: Health Community Inc., 2000.

Stevenson, Lloyd G., and Robert Multhauf, eds. *Medicine, Science, and Culture: Historical Essays in Honor of Owsei Temkin*. Baltimore: Johns Hopkins University Press, 1968.

Stockard, Charles, and George Papanicolaou. "The Existence of a Typical Estrous Cycle in the Guinea Pig; with a Study of Its Histological and Physiological Changes." *American Journal of Anatomy* 7 (1917): 225–83.

Stocker, Midge, ed. *Cancer as a Woman's Issue: Scratching the Surface*. Chicago: Third Side Press, 1991.

Strax, Philip. *The Doctor Talks to You about Breast Cancer*. Hayside, N.Y.: Soundworks, 1975.

———. *Early Detection: Breast Cancer Is Curable*. New York: Harper and Row, 1974.

"Street Fair in View for Needy Patients." *New York Times*, April 23, 1933.

"Surgeons Discuss Cancer Campaign." *Survey*, December 1913, 508–9.

Sutton, J. Bland. *Tumours: Innocent and Malignant: Their Clinical Features and Appropriate Treatment*. Philadelphia: Lea Brothers and Co., 1893.

Sypher, Francis J. "The Rediscovered Prophet: Frederick L. Hoffman (1865–1946)." <http://www.cosmos-club.org/journals/2000/sypher.html>. December 10, 2004.

T. Harkin Department of Defense Appropriation Act, F.Y. 1993. CR 138: S14638–S14643.

Tagliaferri, Mary, Isaac Cohen, and Debu Tripathy, eds. *Breast Cancer: Beyond Convention*. New York: Atria Books, 2002.

Tarkan, Laurie. "A Debate on How to Treat Precancerous Breast Disease." *New York Times*, June 22, 2004.

Temkin, Owsei, ed. *Bulletin of the History of Medicine: Index to Volumes I–XX, 1933–1946*. Baltimore: Johns Hopkins University Press, 1950.

———. *Bulletin of the History of Medicine: Index to Volumes XXI–XXXVI, 1947–1962*. Baltimore: Johns Hopkins University Press, 1966.

Tomes, Nancy. *Gospel of Germs: Men, Women, and the Microbe in American Life*. Cambridge, Mass.: Harvard University Press, 1998.

Treicher, Paula A., Lisa Cartwright, and Constance Penley, eds. *The Visible Woman: Imaging Technologies, Gender, and Science*. New York: New York University Press, 1998.

Trends in Cancer. New York: American Cancer Society, 1965.

"Tribute to Mrs. Rogers." *New York Times*, September 19, 1960.

"Tuberculosis Held Main Harlem Peril." *New York Times*, May 31, 1945.

"The Vanderbilts and the People of Hyde Park." *National Park Service Historical Handbook: Vanderbilt Mansion*. <www.cr.nps.gov/history/online_books/hh/32/hh32i.htm>. December 10, 2004.

Vayena, Eftychia. "Cancer Detectors: An International History of the Pap Test and Cervical Cancer Screening, 1928–1970." Ph.D. diss., University of Minnesota, 1999.

Velpeau, M. *A Treatise of the Diseases of the Breast*. Philadelphia: Carey and Hart, 1841.

"Violet Leaf Treatment of Cancer." *Westminster* 165 (March 1906): 316–19.

Vital Statistics of the United States: 1937, Part 1. Washington, D.C.: Government Printing Office, 1939.

"Volunteer Group Drives on Cancer: 'Women's Field Army' Launches Its Campaign Today with Booths on Public Sites." *New York Times*, March 21, 1937.

Walker, Nancy, ed. *Women's Magazines, 1940–1960*. Boston: Bedford St. Martin's, 1998.

Wangensteen, Owen H., and Sarah D. Wangensteen. *The Rise of Surgery: From Empire Craft to Scientific Discipline*. Minneapolis: University of Minnesota Press, 1978.

"War on Cancer Pressed: Women Are Urged to Enlist in Field Army This Week." *New York Times*, March 22, 1937.

"War on Cancer Pressed: Women Urged to Continue Efforts Despite World Conflict." *New York Times*, October 21, 1943.

Wartic, Nancy, and Julie Felner. "Is Breast Self-Exam Out of Touch?" *Ms.*, November/December 1994, 65–69.

Waserman, Manfred, and Carol Clausen, eds. *Index to Journal of the History of Medicine and Allied Sciences, Volumes I–XXX, 1946–1975*. New Haven, Conn.: n.p., 1977.

Watts, Campbell F., and David M. Elderkin. *Defending the Breast Cancer Malpractice Case*. Englewood Cliffs, N.J.: Prentice Hall Law and Business, 1994.

"We Could Cure Cancer Now!" *Woman's Home Companion*, November 1946, 35, 176.

Weinberg, Robert A. *Racing to the Beginning of the Road: The Search for the Origin of Cancer*. New York: Harmony Books, 1996.

Wells, Mildred White. *Unity in Diversity: The History of the General Federation of Women's Clubs*. Washington, D.C.: General Federation of Women's Clubs, 1953.

Welter, Barbara. "The Cult of True Womanhood: 1820–1860." *American Quarterly* 18 (Summer 1966): 151–74.

"What Is All the Fuss About?" *Time*, February 18, 2002, 53.

White, William Crawford. *Cancer of the Breast*. New York: Harper and Brothers Publishers, 1930.

Whitfield, Steven. *Culture of the Cold War*. Baltimore: Johns Hopkins University, 1991.

Who's Who in America, 1914–1915: A Biographical Dictionary of Notable Living Men and Women of the United States. Chicago: A. N. Marquis and Company, 1914–15.

Who's Who in America: 1938–1939. Chicago: Marquis Company, 1938.

Who Was Who in America, 1897–1942. Vol. 1. Chicago: Marquis, Who's Who, 1966.

"Widen War on Cancer." *New York Times*, February 26, 1939.

Wild, William. "Danger Signals of Cancer." *Hygeia*, December 1926, 699–700.

Wiley, Harvey W. "*If* You *Think* You Have *a Cancer*." *Good Housekeeping*, November 1922, 42, 158–62.

Williams, Ralph Chester. *The United States Public Health Service, 1798–1950*. Washington, D.C.: U.S. Public Health Service, 1951.

"Winning the War against Cancer." *Parents*, June 1973, 49.

"WOMEN NEED NO LONGER DIE of Their No. 1 Cancer Foe." *Ladies' Home Journal*, April 1955, 60–61.

"Women Specialists on Cancer Confer." *New York Times*, March 10, 1944.

"Women's Field Army." *Medical Women's Journal*, February 1938.

Wood, Francis Carter. "Must Women Die of Cancer?" *Woman Citizen* 11 (April 27, 1926): 46–47.

Wright, Louis. "Cancer As It Affects the Negro." *Opportunity*, June 1928, 169–70, 187.

Yalom, Marilyn. *A History of the Breast*. New York: Ballantine Books, 1997.

Zeiss, Genevieve. "A New Life after Breast Cancer." *Ladies' Home Journal*, October 1957, 52–53.

Index

Cytological Diagnostic Conference, 123

Daughters of the American Revolution, 66, 82
Davis, Maxine, 144–45
Day, Emerson, 141–42
Death, 19, 31, 59, 98, 130, 140
Debevoise, Thomas M., 26
De Moulin, Daniel, 7
Denoon, Christopher, 96–97
Domesticity: references to in cancer awareness, 13, 88–89, 117, 150
Downer, Carol, 204
Dyson, W. H., 197

Early detection rhetoric, 2, 5–7, 29, 41, 43, 45, 60, 70, 76, 90–91, 98, 108, 120, 122, 130, 133, 162, 173, 178, 213, 215, 217; individual responsibility and burden of detection, 12, 34, 52, 67, 72, 92, 105, 107, 110, 117, 131, 218
Egan, Robert, 179, 181, 184
Ehrenreich, Barbara, 175, 214–16, 219
Environmental concerns, 7, 8, 220
Erskine, Arthur, 10, 163–73, 247 (nn. 64, 67), 248 (n. 74)
Evans, Sarah, 203

Federation of Colored Women's Clubs, 14, 128–29
Felner, Julie, 219
Female cancers, 10–11, 39
Feminist health movement, 3, 15, 175, 203–4, 208
Films about cancer, 1, 3–5, 9–10, 12, 39, 43–44, 51, 88–91, 104, 122, 124, 127, 131, 133–37, 157, 159, 173, 200–203, 213; *Breast Self-Examination: A Film for Women's Groups*, 10, 116, 118, 130, 134, 160, 163, 214; *The Breast Self-Examination*, 10, 169; *The Great Peril*, 40–42, 48, 120, 228 (n. 77); *Life Saving Fingers*, 111–14, 117, 240 (n. 55); *After Mastectomy*, 152–55; *It's Up to You*, 160–61

Flexner, Marion, 108, 143
Foote, Emerson, 100–103
Ford, Betty, 10, 14, 33, 175–78, 183–84, 186–96, 210; letters of support to, 191–95
Ford, Gerald, 176
Forrester, J. C., 57
Fouty, William, 188–90

Gallup Poll, 130, 160
Gendered references, 5, 6, 18, 29, 41–42, 61, 74, 88–89, 92, 103, 152; and cultural significance of breasts, 13
General Federation of Women's Clubs, 11, 56, 63, 66, 68, 77–78, 82, 157–58, 213; Public Health Division, 70, 71; Cancer Control Fund, 71–72; and WFA, 72–74
Germs: concern about, 18, 41
Gershon-Cohen, Jacob, 179, 181, 184
Government: lobbying, 2, 11, 14, 68, 95, 216–17; politicians, 2, 48, 191; interest in cancer, 7–8, 12, 48, 55, 88–89, 91; Department of Defense, 9; funding, 49, 100; War Department, 49–51
The Great Peril, 40–42, 48, 120, 228 (n. 77)
Greenberg, Daniel, 185

Halsted, William Steward, 21, 22, 28, 55, 164, 165, 188, 196, 198, 214
Height, Dorothy, 158–59
Heredity, 41
Hippocrates, 20
Hoffman, Frederick, 10, 26, 126
Holleb, Arthur, 182
Hope: fostering of in face of cancer, 30, 40, 142, 202
Humoral theory, 20
Huntington, Mrs. Collis P., 79
Huntington Memorial Hospital, 79
Hurdon, Elizabeth, 79
Hygeia, 34
Hysterectomy, 47

United States Public Health Service (USPHS), 48, 88–90, 116, 126, 128, 179, 181, 184, 229 (n. 92)

Vaginal discharge warning, 5, 31, 45, 59, 137, 140, 167
Vaginal smear. *See* Pap smear
Vanderbilt, Louise, 27
Vayena, Eftychia, 121
Virchow, Rudolf, 22

Warning signs of cancer, 5–7, 11, 30–31, 35, 53, 90, 109, 135, 166, 213
Wartic, Nancy, 219
Wiley, Harvey, 32
Wolfson, Sam, 118
Women's clubs: host cancer meetings, 4, 5, 74, 89, 110, 133, 166, 176; and women's space, 9, 14–15, 61, 116, 118; and networks, 11, 19, 53–55, 57, 59, 60, 91; and AAUW, 56, 63–70; and GFWC, 56, 70–72
Women's Field Army (WFA), 12, 53–54, 69–70, 77–87, 91, 95, 124, 136–37, 147, 157; leadership of, 69, 72, 73, 75, 92, 93; membership and recruitment, 74, 76, 78, 90; organization of, 75–76; colored division, 128–29; Iowa, 164, 167
Women's liberation movement, 203–10
Women's networks, informal, 36, 43, 47, 62, 136–37, 172, 219–20
Wood, Susan, 26
Works Progress Administration, 96–97
World's Fair, 160
World War I, 57
World War II, 12–13, 38, 93, 103, 144, 163, 196
Wright, Lois, 127–28

Xerography, 201
X-ray and radiation, 89, 136, 138, 140, 142–43, 164, 166, 171, 179–81, 184

Yolom, Marilyn, 145
Young Women's Christian Association (YWCA), 28, 63, 68, 119, 217

Zonta International, 82